Your symptoms are NOT all in your head!
You may have hypothyroidism.

Are you one of the millions of patients who has been dismissed by doctors because your lab tests were "normal"? Have you been misdiagnosed and unsuccessfully treated with potentially harmful drugs? Don't suffer needlessly anymore! If you answer yes to any of the following, you may have a treatable condition called hypothyroidism.

- Are you always cold, carrying a sweater with you even in the summer?
- Do you have trouble falling asleep or wake suddenly during the night?
- Has your once-shiny hair lost its luster and begun falling out at the slightest touch?
- Does your formerly smooth skin feel rough and dry despite moisturizing?
- Have you noticed that your voice has become deeper or gruffer?
- Are you plagued by head and body aches?
- Are you unable to digest your meals the way you used to?
- Is it hard to recognize the puffy-eyed person in the mirror?
- Has your PMS become more severe?
- Have you maintained your diet but suddenly gained weight?
- Has your once-sharp memory dulled considerably?
- Do you frequently feel depressed and out of sync with the world?

⧂⧂⧂

Despite what some doctors may have told you, you are not doomed to a life of thyroid symptoms. There IS an approach that can work for you—and the millions of others like you.

WHAT YOUR DOCTOR MAY *NOT* TELL YOU ABOUT™

HYPOTHYROIDISM

WHAT YOUR DOCTOR MAY *NOT* TELL YOU ABOUT™

HYPOTHYROIDISM

A Simple Plan for Extraordinary Results

KENNETH BLANCHARD, M.D., PH.D.
with MARIETTA ABRAMS BRILL

WARNER BOOKS

An AOL Time Warner Company

This book is written as a source of information only. It should not substitute for advice from your physician or a qualified health professional. You need to seek the advice of your health care professional before you use any recommendation herein. The authors and the publisher expressly disclaim responsibility for any adverse effects arising from the use of the information in this book.

The case histories included in this book are based on the author's experience with his patients, although their names and personal information have been changed to protect their privacy.

Copyright © 2004 by Ken Blanchard, M.D. and Marietta Abrams Brill
All rights reserved.

The title of the series What Your Doctor May *Not* Tell You About . . . and the related trade dress are trademarks owned by Warner Books and may not be used without permission

Warner Books, Inc., 1271 Avenue of the Americas, New York, NY 10020

Visit our Web site at www.twbookmark.com.

 An AOL Time Warner Company

Printed in the United States of America

First Printing: January 2004
10 9 8 7 6 5 4 3 2 1

Library of Congress Cataloging-in-Publication Data

Blanchard, Kenneth H., M.D.
    What your doctor may not tell you about hypothyroidism : a simple plan for extraordinary results / Kenneth Blanchard, with Marietta Abrams Brill.
        p. cm.
Includes index.
    ISBN 0-446-69061-9
    1. Hypothyroidism—Popular works.   I. Abrams-Brill, Marietta.   II. Title.
RC657.B56 2004
    616.4'44—dc21

                                                                2003052598

Cover design by Diane Lugar
Book design by Charles A. Sutherland

For P.S.B.

—M.A.B.

Acknowledgments

This book exists because of the support of my family and my loyal secretaries over many years: Elizabeth Daniels, Carole Shander, Kay Kearney, Maggie MacLeod, and Betsy Spiro. My practice was helped tremendously by two very splendid laboratory technicians, Barbara Binns and Patty Marsh. The success of my practice since 1996 has been helped immeasurably by the compounding wizardry of Dennis Katz of Hopkinton Drug. Most of all, I thank my many hundreds of patients, who reenergize me every day in the office and who often give me ideas that make the treatment better.

—K.R.B.

Many people created this book. Diana Baroni and Bob Castillo at Warner Books gave it shape and polish. I'm ever grateful to Judith River, my agent, for her encouragement, wise counsel and good humor. Deep gratitude to Karren Abrams, Genia Gould, and Rutha Rosen for their editorial support and friendship, and to the many patients of Dr. Blanchard who courageously shared their stories to help others. For information, I am indebted to many excellent resources including thyroid-info.com (directed by Mary J. Shomon) and the Thyroid Fitness Support Group at Yahoo.com (directed by Charisse Beiswanger, a.k.a. BeeFuddled).

—M.A.B.

Contents

A Note from Dr. Blanchard   xi

Foreword   xiii

PART I HYPOTHYROIDISM: DANGEROUS MEDICAL
         MYTHS, LIFESAVING REVELATIONS   1

Chapter 1. Lifting the Fog on Hypothyroidism   3

Chapter 2. First Stop: Diagnosis   25

Chapter 3. Going Against the Tide: The 2 Percent
              Solution   34

Chapter 4. How I Work with My Patients:
              Translating Theory into Practice   49

Chapter 5. The Tale of the Mouse and the Lizard and
              Other Explanations for Your Symptoms   61

Chapter 6. Who's at Risk for Hypothyroidism?   87

Chapter 7. I Suspect I Have Hypothyroidism
              Because . . .   103

PART II MASTERING YOUR THYROID RHYTHMS AT
          EVERY STAGE OF LIFE   117

Chapter 8. In the Beginning There Was
              Hypothyroidism: Fertility, Pregnancy,
              and Beyond   119

Chapter 9. Giving Your Child the Best Start in
              Infancy and Childhood   134

Chapter 10. Balancing on the Edge: Adolescence
and PMS   147

Chapter 11. It's Also a Guy Thing   156

Chapter 12. Menopause: Finding Your Balance
Amid Change   161

Chapter 13. Keeping the Beat in Advanced Age   173

PART III THE CARE AND FEEDING OF THE AILING
THYROID   181

Chapter 14. Is Hypothyroidism in the Air?   185

Chapter 15. What You Should Know About
Weight Gain and Hypothyroidism   193

Chapter 16. Dr. Blanchard's Thyroid Wellness Diet 199

Chapter 17. Ten Hazards of Healthy Living:
Holistic Habits That Could Make
You More Hypo   212

Chapter 18. Top Tips from Dr. Blanchard's
Patients (Plus a Few More)   216

Chapter 19. Finding a Doctor You Can Talk to—
and Doing It Effectively   223

Resources   227
Glossary   233
Index   247

A Note from Dr. Blanchard

A very common ritual experienced by many medical students at the end of their years in medical school is to hear an address by an eminent medical dean, who congratulates them and wishes them well in their internships, then says something like this: "Half of what you learned in medical school is wrong, and your challenge now is to find out which half." This may sound whimsical, but it does reflect a very basic truth about the complexity of the human body and immensity of medical knowledge. It is also often said that the only people who are 100 percent sure about anything in medicine are medical students, malpractice lawyers, and well-compensated expert witnesses. In my opinion, much of the "factual knowledge" that has been taught to physicians about hypothyroidism falls into the "wrong" category, so that the original title of this work was "The Many Myths of Hypothyroidism." It is my deep belief that the current status of the TSH test as the absolute yes-or-no arbiter for the presence of hypothyroidism and for the status of a patient's treatment will eventually come to be regarded as one of the great mistakes of medical history.

Foreword

—— •◆• ——

What won't your doctor tell you about hypothyroidism? Unfortunately, most doctors won't tell you very much at all about this common but frequently overlooked condition.

One thing your doctor may not tell you—or even be aware of—is the difficult situation many hypothyroid patients face in even getting diagnosed. The incidence of hypothyroidism is vastly underestimated. During the past fifteen years, experts have changed their estimates from fewer than 5 million, to 8 million to 12 million, to as many as 20 million or more Americans affected. Hypothyroidism is also vastly undiagnosed. Symptoms can sometimes be vague or can mimic many other conditions, making diagnosis difficult. The bottom line: Millions of you are hypothyroid, and many millions more of you are hypothyroid but don't know yet or may never know.

What else won't your doctor tell you about hypothyroidism? Your doctor isn't likely to tell you that the thyroid hormone replacement drug you will probably receive—synthetic thyroxine, known as levothyroxine, *l*-thyroxine, or T4—is a standard, cookie-cutter treatment given to most patients. And chances are that this standard treatment won't be enough to restore your optimal health.

Another thing your doctor may not tell you is what will happen if you still don't feel well after being treated. When you bring up unresolved symptoms and health complaints, you may be written off as a "mental case" and given antidepressants or packed off to see the psychiatrist. Or you may be told you're lazy and that the solution to your fatigue or weight gain is simply to "get off the couch, get moving, and stop eating so much." And, because hypothyroidism affects women much more than men, many of you will be dismissed as "hormonal," suffering from PMS, experiencing "postpartum blues," or being in menopause, and given prescriptions for hormones, the pill, or more antidepressants.

What your doctor also may not tell you is that an apparent mob psychology rules the mainstream diagnosis and treatment process with an iron fist. And it's been this way for quite a long time. Changes in thyroid treatment seem to move at a glacial pace. The standard operating procedure—TSH test, followed by treatment with levothyroxine—is not only the same today as it was when I was first diagnosed with hypothyroidism in 1995, but it's been the same for thirty years.

I'll admit it sounds somewhat dire. Are there any doctors out there who *will* help you get diagnosed and feel better?

Absolutely.

There are a few innovative, independent, courageous, patient-oriented doctors who have led the charge for better hypothyroidism treatment. Doctors who asserted all along that undiagnosed hypothyroidism was reaching epidemic proportions . . . Doctors who were unfazed by the marketing pitches for synthetic thyroxine and continued to successfully prescribe the less expensive natural dessiccated thyroid drugs that had been working well all along for their patients . . . Doctors who knew that unresolved symptoms in thyroid patients could not just be written off to depression, stress, or PMS, and found real solutions instead . . . Doctors who continued to rely on clinical examination, observation, family history, and tests to make a diagnosis of hypothyroidism, refusing to succumb to what Dr. John Lowe calls "the tyranny of the TSH test" . . . Doctors who recognized early that there were reasons why patients did not feel well on the conventional levothyroxine therapy and available solutions.

These doctors have bucked convention—often on the receiving end of the raised eyebrows of their medical colleagues—in order to restore caring and common sense to the process of diagnosing and treating hypothyroidism.

Dr. Kenneth Blanchard is a standout among this small group of pioneers, a leader in the effort to humanize hypothyroidism treatment.

I first became aware of his work when I started my Thyroid Top Doctors Directory at my Web site. Recommendations were flying in from patients of Dr. Blanchard, nominating him as a Thyroid Top Doc and reporting on their success at regaining energy, sex drive, lost hair, and resolution of other symptoms.

When I sat down in 1999 to decide which practitioners to interview when writing my own thyroid book, *Living Well with Hypothyroidism*, Dr. Blanchard was on the list. It was at that time that I had the great pleasure to get to know him, interview him at length, learn more about his innovative ideas about thyroid treatment, and feature his work in my book.

In addition to his innovative ideas, it was a pleasure for me, as a patient advocate, to discover a physician who so truly understood and shared the aims, objective, and philosophy of the patients he treated.

Dr. Blanchard and I share a common frustration for people who have family histories of thyroid disease and who had thyroid symptoms (fatigue, weight changes, hair loss, enlarged thyroid, nodules, etc.) but whose TSH tests were in the low or high end of normal and were sent away by doctors without diagnosis or treatment. We have frequently talked about how unfortunate it is that this narrow-minded and near-slavish reliance on the TSH test—often to the exclusion of clinical evidence—has been the "standard of care" for conventional doctors and endocrinologists for decades.

Dr. Blanchard and I also share a certainty that the TSH test is just one factor among many that can aid in a diagnosis of hypothyroidism—and should not be a sole arbiter of diagnosis. This becomes particularly important in light of the current reevaluation of the reference range for what is considered even "normal" TSH-wise.

Many physicians and drug manufacturers believe that hypothyroidism is "easy to treat." "One pill a day takes care of everything," they cavalierly tell patients. But Dr. Blanchard has stood with our patient community as we have fought against that myth.

Conventional endocrinologists have frequently chosen to dismiss or overlook a growing body of evidence, both anecdotal and empirical, that shows that patients need more than levothyroxine to feel well. In fact, several years ago, I conducted the first large-scale quality-of-life survey among thyroid patients, with more than one thousand participants. More than 50 percent of respondents reported that they did not feel well and were not satisfied with their thyroid treatment. A Thyroid Foundation of America survey in the late 1990s found that more than two-thirds of Graves' disease patients continued to suffer debilitating symptoms after treatment. And Drs. Prange and Bunevicius and their colleagues who participated in the groundbreaking research reported in the *New England Journal of Medicine* in February 1999 offered in mainstream medical literature an explanation for why patients did not feel well. This landmark study found that the majority of thyroid patients studied felt better on a combination of two drugs that provided both thyroxine (T4) and triiodothyronine (T3), NOT solely T4. The conventional, standard treatment with levothyroxine-only products is not the best approach for the majority of patients.

Dr. Blanchard has been one of the few physicians to speak out against the levothyroxine-only conventional dogma and argue for more comprehensive treatment for patients. He has been working with supplemental T3 for years and has had an opportunity to treat smart, empowered, and outspoken patients. Working as a true partner of these patients, Dr. Blanchard has been able to help them find the optimal balance of T4 and T3 that allows them to feel their absolute best. Along the way, the knowledge he has gained has allowed him to fine-tune the approach he uses to help his hypothyroid patients achieve optimal wellness.

It is the benefit of his years of experience—and the experiences of the patients who have flourished under his care—that Dr. Blanchard brings us to in this book, grounded in common sense, open-mindedness, and compassion for patients.

Ken Blanchard is the doctor many thyroid patients wish they had—a conventionally trained and educated physician who has shown he was willing to listen to his patients when they told him that what he learned in medical school might not be working for them. He looked for solutions, and he found them. He was not satisfied to pull out his endocrinology textbook from the 1970s and declare that it contains all there is to know about thyroid disease. Instead, he delved in, figured things out, and has never stopped learning. By trusting his own instincts and listening to his patients, he learns something new every day about how to best diagnose and treat hypothyroidism.

As a thyroid patient advocate, I am thrilled that Dr. Blanchard's book has been published, because we need every voice we can in the effort to raise awareness of thyroid disease. And I am even more thrilled that his book so effectively demonstrates how innovative thyroid treatment approaches—not canned, formulaic solutions—are the real answer for the millions of people with hypothyroidism.

Those of us in the thyroid patient community are fortunate that Dr. Ken Blanchard has taken this opportunity to share his wealth of experience with us in *What Your Doctor May Not Tell You About Hypothyroidism.*

Mary J. Shomon
March 2003
Kensington, MD

MARY J. SHOMON is a patient advocate and author of the books *Living Well with Hypothyroidism: What Your Doctor Doesn't Tell You . . . That You Should Know* and *Living Well with Autoimmune Disease: What Your Doctor Doesn't Tell You . . . That You Should Know.* She also manages the Web site www.thyroid-info.com and edits several patient newsletters.

PART I

Hypothyroidism:
Dangerous Medical Myths,
Lifesaving Revelations

Chapter 1

· ◆ ·

Lifting the Fog on Hypothyroidism

FROM HERE TO OBSCURITY

Maybe you can remember it—a time when your energy and capacity were in sync with your life. Think back and recapture that sense of moving with relative ease through the world. Your energy flowed with the pace set by night and day. During the day, your physical and mental powers were at your service, while nighttime brought the restful sleep needed for energetic days—and the cycle repeated. You ate in proportion to your needs, without unexpected changes in weight. For the most part (heredity notwithstanding), your hair stayed where it belonged—on your head instead of the shower floor. If you are a woman, you experienced the normal ups and downs of life's cycles: puberty, menstruation, fertility, menopause.

Aside from the normal changes in life, your outlook was generally positive.

Then slowly, over time, you began to lose step. A mix of symptoms, ranging from subtle to incapacitating, burden you.

3

Now you are unable to keep up. You probably feel cold more often. You're the one who always needs to take a sweater to a restaurant in the summer. For many of you, seasonal and hormonal changes upset your internal rhythms and send your symptoms into overdrive. You feel drained of energy, and all you want to do is stay in bed, but a good night's sleep is just a dream. Insomnia and sudden wakings disrupt your sleep. Not only has your hair lost its luster, but it is brittle and falling out at the faintest touch. Your skin feels rough and dry. The area around your eyes looks puffy, and your voice has deepened or become gruffer. You get muscle cramps, and your reflexes are weak. Headaches, body aches/joint pain, low blood sugar, constipation and other digestive problems, severe PMS, unexplained weight gain—these symptoms may have cropped up. If you are a woman, your periods might have become heavier and longer, or they have disappeared altogether. Then there are the emotional and mental effects. The color seems to have seeped out of your life, and your memory has slipped. You are no longer nearly as social as you once were, which adds to your sense of being out of step with the world. You are depressed (who wouldn't be?) and emotionally unsteady.

In short, you have symptoms of hypothyroidism.

KEEPING PACE WITH LIFE'S CHANGE

Like a flawless dance partner, thyroid hormones are highly sensitive to changes in your ever-changing environment. They take the lead in setting the metabolic pace, helping you adapt to changes in temperature, stress, hormonal fluctuations, and other conditions.

When there are ample amounts of thyroid hormone doing the rounds, the body is more apt to respond in a realistic and healthy way to changes. When thyroid levels are low, the body slows down, lost in a fog of sensory stimuli that it cannot detect, much less respond to.

More scientifically speaking, researchers and clinicians know that the hormones produced by the thyroid, called T4 and T3, are architects of the body's ever-shifting metabolism. Metabolism is the use of oxygen and nutrients by cells to make energy. Generally, the higher your metabolism, the more energetic you feel (when metabolism's too high, you might feel "hyper"). When your metabolism flags, though, so does your physical and mental vigor.

THE HYPOTHYROID FOG

Certainly, no single person has all of the symptoms described above. Each individual is unique. Chances are your suite of symptoms differs from another's. Yet underlying almost everyone's symptoms is what many weary patients describe as "brain fog": Your energy is zapped, and with it you have lost your memory, your capacity to think clearly, the color in your life, your personality. As one of my patients described it, it feels as though someone stuffed cotton between your ears. You are essentially robbed of your inspiration, your passion, and your ability to live a full live.

When the hypothyroid fog sets in, the strong, vital internal metronome that once drove your life forward in sync with your life's distinctive melody—with all the high notes and low notes that went along with it—has been muted.

The fog is not just a pervasive symptom; it is an apt metaphor for the state of hypothyroidism treatment today. This fog has infiltrated the minds and lives of an estimated 27 million patients, yet only about 75 percent of people with a depleted thyroid are diagnosed, and many are not adequately treated.

WHAT DOCTORS MAY *NOT* TELL YOU . . . BECAUSE THEY DO NOT KNOW

Much of what you read in this book will probably be new to you. You might assume that your doctor certainly would have tried this approach, or at least told you about it. The fact is that your doctor may not know about my approach—or any other that deviates from his or her knowledge. Too often, physicians follow the conventions of their field and never look to see what might work better. I developed this method based on what I learned in medical school and then what I learned from my patients. I observed them closely and studied what works, then adjusted therapy accordingly. Everything I do would be approved by the Food and Drug Administration, and there are many articles in well-regarded medical journals that support my concepts. However, in spite of the growing demand for new approaches and the groundswell of information supporting them, too few doctors seem to pay attention. As a result, most doctors hold close the three tenets of treatment for hypothyroidism that have left many patients suffering.

Three Flaws in the Conventional Approach to Hypothyroidism

In my view, there are three serious flaws with the conventional approach to hypothyroidism:

1. Conventional medicine bases diagnosis on a test that does not detect all patients. The only certain way to diagnose hypothyroidism is with a trial of thyroid that is fine-tuned to patient response.
2. Mainstream doctors endorse only one treatment: the synthetic thyroid hormone T4. If you continue to feel poorly, most doctors will tell you that your symptoms have another cause, because "you are on a thyroid medicine and your test

numbers are good." They seldom make use of other highly effective options: T3 and natural thyroid extract.
3. When it *is* employed, T3 is rarely used in the right proportion.

In more than two decades of treating hypothyroidism, I have seen these mistakes over and over in patients who come to me looking for confirmation that their symptoms have a cause, and looking for a way to end years of misery. As a result, I've come to see hypothyroidism in a different light than my conventional colleagues do.

I believe in my patient first and foremost. Symptoms and patient history are far better indicators of disease than the TSH test. After twenty-five years of judicious trial and error, I've seen thousands and thousands of patients respond immensely well to physiologic proportions of T3 and T4: 2 percent T3 and 98 percent T4. My 2 percent solution.

WHY I WROTE THIS BOOK

It may seem simple and obvious to treat patients as individuals and to use all of the therapeutic tools available. But my approach, though rooted in common sense and the best of today's clinical knowledge, is virtually unknown by the vast majority of hypothyroid patients and their clinicians. That's why I felt compelled to write *What Your Doctor May* Not *Tell You About Hypothyroidism.*

This book was written for the individuals who are looking for a simple, clinically safe, and patient-proven way to end their symptoms. For the first time in any book, you will find a description of how hypothyroidism affects individuals—

women *and* men—at every life stage. You'll also find how my treatment helps where others have failed, both in my words and in the words of my patients.

This book was written for the millions of people whose symptoms have been dismissed by other doctors because their lab tests were "normal"—and who were misdiagnosed and treated, often unnecessarily, for other conditions with potentially harmful drugs. All the while their hypothyroidism and its symptoms continue untreated, contributing to fatigue, weight gain, and potentially dangerous heart problems—to name just a few. This book will give you hope that your symptoms are not all in your head. You are not doomed to a lifetime of thyroid symptoms because there *is* an approach that works for you—and for the millions of others like you.

Last but not least, I wrote this book for open-minded physicians who have sensed that the conventional approach may work for some patients, but not for all, and are looking for a new tactic. Herein you will find the clinical rationale behind my approach, and a clear step-by-step outline of my strategy. My unique 2 percent T3 solution has allowed me to help thousands of patients. It is my hope that it will give doctors the tools to effectively treat millions more.

KEEPING UP WITH THE TIMES

Importantly, thyroid rhythms change over time with our bodies' metabolic needs. Our bodies and environments are in constant flux. It is the job of the thyroid and related endocrine (hormonal) system to be exquisitely sensitive to changes in the body's internal and external environment and to help our bodies keep a metabolic balance that accommodates these changes. As the body's needs change, so does its need for thyroid hormone. The challenge is finding a good match and continually fine-tuning treatment to changing rhythms. I am honored that my patients' health is the most convincing testimony to this alternative approach. Michelle is one example.

The term "slow motion" is the last one Michelle would use to describe herself. She is a fit and glowing mother of three children and the director/teacher of a thriving yoga center. But those are the words she used to describe her life before discovering yoga and receiving my thyroid treatment.

When she first came to see me at the age of thirty-nine, Michelle was overweight and mentally foggy, and she suffered from insomnia. Her face was swollen, and she had terrible acne. In our first input session, Michelle traced her symptoms back to her teenage years—as so many of my patients do! She remembered often feeling lethargic and depressed. She was formally diagnosed as hypothyroid at the age of eighteen based on a high level of thyroid-stimulating hormone (TSH).

By the time she was thirty, Michelle was diagnosed with Hashimoto's autoimmune thyroiditis, the most common cause of hypothyroidism. Severe headaches had led her to neurologists who identified a venous stricture in her brain. Another neurologist diagnosed epilepsy; she subsequently experienced a toxic reaction to antiseizure medications. Just a few in a long, long decade of "worse and worse stories," culminating in the prospect of a brain surgery, thyroidectomy (removal of the thyroid gland), and exploratory surgery on her colon.

Then two events changed her life: yoga and effective thyroid treatment. With yoga, Michelle immediately felt the mental fog lift, and she slept better—the beginning of her road to wellness. "The other part of the equation was Dr. Blanchard," she says, whom she discovered through the Web site of Mary J. Shomon, thyroid patient advocate and published educator, at www.thyroid-info.com.

As is customary, I took a complete history. Based on Michelle's symptoms, my recommendation was a combination of natural thyroid extract (Armour) and levothyroxine (Synthroid), also known as T4. My aim with Michelle was to replace the missing thyroid hormone in *physiologic doses*—that is, a dosage to restore a healthy balance of thyroid hormones. A short trial with my regimen quickly uncovered a problem: skin irritations and outbreaks. Many people with Hashimoto's thyroiditis have multiple immunologic problems, including allergies. The skin problems cleared up when I switched Michelle to a dye-free dosage form of Synthoid. "Other doctors would have sent me to a dermatologist," says Michelle.

Michelle relies on me to keep the chemistry in balance, and she balances out with yoga. Together we make a good team.

Because our bodies are constantly changing, I encourage all of my patients to stay tuned to changes in their symptoms and to let me know about them so that I can make the necessary dosage adjustments. "For me, the first things to go are my digestive system, sleep patterns, and mental clarity," Michelle says. "I'm sensitive to even slight changes," which she takes as warnings for a change in dosage.

Over the course of six months, Michelle went from a woman not living up to her potential to a woman embracing and acting on her abilities. The impact on her family, her marriage, and her professional life has been enormous. Today she is symptom-free and able to live her life fully.

Many of my patients have learned to take their symptoms seriously and insist that their doctors do the same. I encourage my patients to be *active partners in their treatment*. It is my hope that this book will instill a similar sense of confidence and empowerment in my readers—to give them the confidence to trust their feelings and to persist in finding a doctor who gives them the same level of respect.

Most doctors would probably have never given Michelle thyroid treatment, because her tests were normal. If she had followed the recommendations of various specialists, she may have been misdiagnosed and ended up with unneeded treatments, a shunt in her brain or a double bowel resection, while her hypothyroidism persisted, untreated or poorly treated with 100 percent T4.

As this and many other cases show, what you don't know about hypothyroidism can hurt you. This is a critical lesson that we'll explore in more detail throughout this book, so that you will have the knowledge to seek out an accurate diagnosis and the treatment you need.

WHAT DOCTORS MAY *NOT* TELL YOU ABOUT DIAGNOSIS

The American Academy of Clinical Endocrinologists (AACE) is the governing body for endocrinologists, the doctors who specialize in hormone problems like hypothyroidism. Over the past two years, they have twice revised the ranges considered normal for thyroid function. Basically, they continue to expand the lab test range for the TSH to include more patients with hypothyroidism. According to a 2003 AACE press release, "The prevalence of undiagnosed thyroid disease is shockingly high, particularly since it is a condition that is easy to diagnose and treat."

It's great that doctors are being encouraged to test more often and to heighten their awareness of hypothyroidism. The unfortunate fact is that diagnoses will continue to be missed by most physicians when they base it solely on their recommended "easy to diagnose" testing method, rather than on how the patient feels.

TSH Tests: The Good, the Bad, and the Irrelevant

As far as tests go, the TSH is a very accurate (in lab-ese, "sensitive") test for what it is designed to measure: thyroid-stimulating hormone. Doctors can feel confident that it will do what it should. The problem is how the results are used.

Depending on the laboratory, most physicians suspect hypo-thyroidism if the TSH levels are *above* the normal range. This range is based on guidelines from the AACE and other governing organizations. TSH levels that are higher than a certain level indicate hypothyroidism. TSH levels *below* a certain level are considered normal or, when even lower, *hyper*thyroid.

Specifically, as of February 2003, the AACE encourages doctors to treat patients who test outside the boundaries of a target TSH level of 0.3 to 3.4 uU/ml. Mary J. Shomon, hypothyroid patient advocate, author of *Living Well with Hypothyroidism* (see page 228), and editor of the highly informative Web site www.thyroid-info.com, encapsulates the situation like this:

Until November 2002, people who had clear symptoms of thyroid disease, but were in the normal range on the TSH scale, were considered "euthyroid" or normal by almost all endocrinologists and practitioners, and were *not* diagnosed at all, much less easily diagnosed. People who had family histories of thyroid disease, symptoms (including enlarged thyroid, goiter, nodules, etc.), but whose TSH tests were in the low or high end of normal were routinely denied treatment or told that their problems were the result of depression and given antidepressants. This has gone on for decades, as conventional medicine has relied on the TSH test—often to the exclusion of clinical evidence, symptoms, and medical observation—to make a diagnosis. I would not consider this evidence of "easy to diagnose," particularly from the perspective of the millions of patients who have suffered with undiagnosed thyroid disease, not to mention the suffering that resulted from being misdiagnosed with a host of mental or physical ailments by their doctors and prescribed various drugs, hormones, and other inappropriate treatments.

High TSH Means Low Thyroid Levels

I know that it sounds strange that a higher-than-normal blood test indicates lower-than-normal thyroid function. That's because the TSH is a measure not of thyroid hormone itself, but of a hormone that stimulates the thyroid to produce thyroid hormones.

Thyroid hormone levels low in the blood
↓
TSH levels high
↓
Thyroid gland produces more thyroid hormone

In effect, the TSH aims to reflect the *need* for thyroid hormone in the blood. A high TSH indicates a high level of *depletion*. As we'll see in chapter 2, the TSH test does not always accurately reflect thyroid status. I'll go into more detail about these hormones later on in the book.

I use the TSH as a more individualized marker for the success of treatment, but not as the sole basis for diagnosis. Indeed, many of my patients can cite their "personal" TSH—the level where they feel best. But as I mentioned, in some patients the test is completely irrelevant.

The TSH "normal" range is determined by measuring TSH levels in large numbers of "normal" individuals. Plotting these results on a graph gives a bell-shaped curve. By statistical formulas, a few percentage points on the shoulder of the curve on each side are chopped off, giving the "normal" range. It is important to note that a lab result represents a range, not an absolute. In addition, the normal range for thyroid function is very broad, as far as ranges go. Many confirmed cases of hypothyroidism were not diagnosed sooner simply because the individuals' tests were normal—even when patients didn't *feel* normal.

The question in my mind is always this: At what TSH level do my patients feel best? My measure of success is my patient's well-being, not his or her test numbers.

The Tragic Consequences of Undiagnosed Hypothyroidism

As Michelle's case showed all too clearly, having symptoms of hypothyroidism with a normal TSH result sends many patients off on the convoluted path of medical specialists.

If you were depressed, you were probably referred to a psychiatrist. Aches and pains: a rheumatologist. Migraines? A neurologist. Extreme fatigue: a psychologist, allergist. Constipation? Gastroenterologist. *Hypothyroidism is rarely on the radar of these specialists,* who by definition focus on the body system that they know best. You might have managed to get some symptom relief, but with the underlying cause persisting, new and potentially life-threatening problems are bound to crop up.

Consider Jackie. At age fifty-one she had lost the better part of her vital adult life to undiagnosed hypothyroidism:

Depending on the symptom, the specialist would recommend a treatment in that area. I had swelling in my feet and tarsal tunnel syndrome, and the podiatrist wanted to operate on me. The orthopedist said I had sympathetic dystrophy. An ear, nose, and throat specialist told me I had TMJ. I went from doctor to doctor. Depression landed me with three different antidepressants. I do have antithyroid antibodies, but they weren't even measured until I finally "proved" myself to an endocrinologist with a TSH of 6.0!

If only the problem ended with an accurate diagnosis.

WHAT DOCTORS MAY *NOT* TELL YOU ABOUT TREATMENT

Doctors will tell you that treatment is also straightforward. The missing thyroid hormone is replaced in pill form, usually as a pure synthetic form of T4 called levothyroxine. Once the body has the hormone it needs, you should feel well.

What they will not tell you is that, with this single-minded treatment plan, patients are inadequately treated, even when measured by the conventional TSH test. According to the Colorado Thyroid Disease Prevalence Study of more than 25,000 people, reported in the February 2000 issue of the *Archives of Internal Medicine*, in spite of treatment, TSH levels were abnormal in 40 percent of those who were hypothyroid.

In the first large-scale quality-of-life survey of hypothyroid patients (710 patients), conducted by Mary J. Shomon, 50 percent reported that they are not satisfied with their treatment. (Read more at www.thyroid.about.com.)

T4 Is a Misleading Treatment Option

T4 is one of two major active hormones produced by the thyroid gland; the other is T3. (There are others as well, which will be discussed in chapter 2.) For many years, doctors used natural thyroid extract, made from animal thyroid, to treat hypothyroidism. Then pharmaceutical research found a way to reproduce pure T4 synthetically. Today it is the mainstay of treatment for hypothyroidism.

Synthetic T4 comes under the brand names of Levoxyl, Unithroid, Synthroid, and Levothroid. It is true that T4 often works beautifully for a short period, or if patients are lucky, longer. But symptoms commonly creep back, while blood tests remain normal. Now the patient is in double trouble. At this point, many doctors argue that the original diagnosis was incorrect, bringing the frustrated (and symptom-plagued) patient back to square one. Many of these patients end up at my door. The medical profession casts a jaundiced eye on any plan that departs from this single-minded strategy.

The Body Needs More Than T4.

T4 is just one of several known hormones produced by the thyroid gland. The thyroid also makes T3 (the more active hormone) and purportedly inactive hormones such as the T1s and T2s. So why do most doctors tell you that you only need T4? Medical doctrine has it that T4 converts to T3 in the body's tissues. Doctors are taught that if T4 converts to T3 and other Ts, then there's no reason to replace thyroid hormones other than T4.

It is my strong belief, and that of a growing number of other clinicians, that many factors can cause clinical hypothyroidism, not just inadequate production of T4.

The thyroid itself produces T3, albeit in much smaller quantities than T4. Some researchers assert that certain organ tissues, like those in the brain, need the thyroid-direct form of T3 to function, not just the T3 made by conversion in the tissue. I'll discuss this in more detail in chapter 3. As a result, based on theory and my experience with thousands of patients, I strongly believe that people with hypothyroidism also need T3 treatment and probably the other Ts as well.

But T3 has many detractors. They point to studies showing that T3 is not effective. That it can cause palpitations (racing heartbeat). They say that it doesn't last long in the body, making it necessary to take multiple inconvenient doses.

THE 2 PERCENT SOLUTION: A SOLUTION BASED ON WHAT WORKS IN PATIENTS

It is true. The correct dosing of T3 is important in order to achieve effectiveness and to avoid side effects. Having prescribed T3 in one form or another for more than fifteen years, I have arrived at a dose that reflects the natural balance of hormones in a healthy thyroid system—what I term a physiologic balance. I call it the 2 percent solution.

Thousands of Patients Can't Be Wrong

The 2 percent solution is based on treating thousands of patients in my practice who were suffering on T4 alone. It's the result of years of fine-tuning treatment to arrive at a physiologic dose of T3 and T4. Over time, I began to see a pattern of success: Patients responded beautifully when the dose proportion was 2 percent T3 and 98 percent T4.

This 98:2 proportion can be achieved with either synthetic hormones (using a time-release capsule for T3) or natural thyroid extract. Many of my patients respond wonderfully to this proportion with natural desiccated thyroid extract (Armour). Armour contains roughly 80 percent T4 and 20 percent T3. By adding the right amount of synthetic T4, I arrive at the natural physiologic balance.

Of course, there will always be a small number of patients who do fine on 100 percent synthetic T4. And I am very happy to continue prescribing it. But for the majority of patients who don't do well on T4, there's immense relief in having a new therapeutic option that works.

The improvements with this combination have been called lifesaving by my patients because of the many ways they experience relief: Years of fatigue lift. Skin moistens. Depression disappears. Headaches evaporate. After years of debilitation, my patients can function wholly again.

Consider again the case of Jackie. When we left her earlier, she was shuttling from specialist to specialist:

I'd heard about Dr. Blanchard from Mary Shomon's Web site at About.com. So I wrote him a letter telling him my story, and he agreed to see me. He put me on a time-release form of T3 with T4, and I couldn't believe it. Within two days the fog had lifted. There is no way to describe it—to me it was a miracle. I guess I'm lucky in the sense that hypothyroidism is a disease that can improve quickly when you have the right treatment. I consider myself lucky to have gotten better—and to have been given the right tool to keep myself well.

KEEPING UP WITH LIFE'S CHANGES: THE HYPOTHYROID CHALLENGE

The thyroid is an instrument of change. As the master of the body's metabolism, the healthy thyroid helps the body adapt without much fuss to minute-by-minute, climate-driven, seasonal, and life-stage changes. As you read this, your thyroid is busy at work helping you adjust to changes in temperature, stress levels, the food you ate for lunch.

In treating thousands of patients over the years, I've seen that symptoms peak and wane with seasonal, metabolic, and hormonal shifts, and sometimes these changes are great enough to warrant a change in treatment. It's not unusual for symptoms to return when the seasons change—or for new symptoms to appear when patients enter different life stages (which we'll look at more closely in part II).

- Childhood. The body's constant growth puts an exceptionally high demand on the metabolic and hormonal systems. Symptoms and signs of hypothyroidism such as short stature, irritability, difficulty in concentrating, and/or ADD can be either easily ignored or misdiagnosed, leading to the prescribing of potentially dangerous medications. If symptoms point to hypothyroidism and tests are normal, I would recommend a trial of thyroid medication. This is safer and more "diagnostic" than administering mood-altering drugs or such agents as Ritalin.

- Puberty. Shifting hormones can wreak havoc on a thyroid-deprived endocrine system. Are the symptoms of PMS—constipation/diarrhea, cold intolerance, headaches, cramps—due to normal hormonal fluctuations or hypothyroidism? If there is a family history, I certainly consider a trial of thyroid replacement, especially when over-the-counter medications fail.

- Infertility. Inability to conceive, miscarriage, and pregnancy complications may be a woman's first indication of hypothyroidism. It may cause anovulation (failure to ovulate), short luteal phase (the time between ovulation and onset of menstrual flow), and other problems. The demands for thyroid hormone during the time of conception are higher than normal, so patients with borderline/low thyroid function may have problems conceiving. For women already diagnosed with hypothyroidism, as well as those suspecting it due to infertility, I recommend trials of thyroid replacement and close monitoring.

- Pregnancy. Pregnancy causes a sudden rise in thyroid hormone needs, as much is diverted to the maturing embryo. If a patient's symptoms have been well controlled on thyroid medication and she suddenly experiences symptoms, a thyroid checkup is in order. Undertreated hypothyroidism can result in a learning problem, or even a lower IQ, in the child later. I tune thyroid levels to my patients' symptoms rather than the TSH.

- Menopause. The change in life creates a hormonal roller coaster. The educated woman will know that estrogen replacement is often considered a panacea for menopausal symptoms; that it is important to clarify whether symptoms are due to hypothyroidism or estrogen depletion; and that a carefully individualized regimen of estrogen, thyroid, progesterone, and possibly other hormones is required to achieve a healthy balance during this time.

- Advanced age. At a certain point, as with other body systems, the thyroid begins to slow down. An estimated 20 percent of women over the age of sixty have hypothyroidism. I discuss hormonal changes and examine symptoms closely with patients who may need extra supplementation at the time when their body's natural supply wanes.

- Weight gain is often blamed on thyroid deficiency, which may be the case. But unfortunately, the remedy is not always thyroid replacement. Close attention to diet, especially one that synchronizes with natural metabolic rhythms, is most effective.

- Seasonal changes. In addition to hormonal shifts, seasonal changes impose variations in response to treatment and may trigger changes in the emotional and physical health of my patients. These observations make perfect sense considering the role of thyroid hormones in regulating metabolism. (See page 61.)

MY OWN STORY

I started my career as an endocrinologist with the same doctrinaire approach to hypothyroidism as my colleagues. I performed the TSH test when symptoms indicated, and treated only when the tests indicated an abnormality. My break from medical orthodoxy began in 1985, when a young female patient came to see me with an article from a popular health magazine. That article claimed that symptoms of premenstrual syndrome are due to thyroid deficiency, a concept that is still unaccepted by conventional doctors.

I never treated that patient because her TSH tests for hypothyroidism were negative—and I was not ready to defy medical convention yet. But the experience was eye-opening. Little did I know then that this one patient would come to represent a turning point in my professional life, and in the lives of thousands of men and women I have since successfully treated for hypothyroidism. Over the next few years, I began tentatively

treating patients whose TSH tests indicated borderline hypothyroidism, and I was surprised by the positive response. The
successes I experienced gave me the courage to extend my clinical reach to individuals with symptoms strongly suggestive of
hypothyroidism, irrespective of their TSH results.

Over time, I also began exploring unorthodox uses of available treatments—all approved, but some only rarely used, such
as T3 in combination with T4. Through observation of my patients, the seasonal and hormonal patterns I described above
began to emerge.

I have refined my approach over the past decade. The result
is a system rooted in several simple ideas that were conceived
by observation, pursued by intuition, and proved by cautious,
empirical treatment of thousands of my patients.

First and foremost, *I listen to patients' symptoms, not necessar-
ily the lab results.* As I've explained, the patient's presentation is
more telling than any test. I routinely use a combination of the
two to make clinical decisions.

Second, *I balance thyroid levels by administering "physiologic"
doses of hormones according to the 2 percent solution.* Not only is
hypothyroidism often underdiagnosed, but even after diagnosis it's usually poorly treated. As stated earlier, my therapeutic
aim is to reproduce the body's normal balance of T3 and T4
through physiologic (not pharmacologic) doses of these two
hormones—doses that reflect an individual's body in health. In
my experience, that proportion is 2 percent T3 and 98 percent
T4. This solution has worked for many thousands of my patients. However, it often requires more than one visit to
achieve the right balance. In the following chapters, you will
discover the medical rationale behind T4/T3 treatment, sce-
narios where different treatments are successfully used, and
how to broach the subject of this effective but unconventional
treatment with your own doctor.

People are dynamic beings and thyroid needs change. So should treatment. It is imperative to *tune thyroid levels to changing life rhythms.* Some people can hum along for years taking the same prescription with no problem but then, suddenly, with a change in conditions, symptoms flare up. Puberty, pregnancy, menopause, seasonal changes, times of great physical or emotional stress—all can throw hormones off balance. I will help you to understand why certain milestones in the life cycle disrupt hormonal rhythms and how to recognize these changes in yourself, and I will give you some pointers for discussing with your doctor the need for adjustments.

Reduce weight with a solid nutritional and exercise plan. Many people with hypothyroidism are aware of difficulties in losing excess weight. A slower metabolism, lower energy levels, and depression—these are symptoms of hypothyroidism that conspire to add pounds. Because you're using less energy, you do need fewer calories than people with normal thyroid function. But that's only when your thyroid is functioning on low. Thyroid hormone replacement will *not* solve weight problems—it will only level the playing field so that you have the energy to exercise and take more active control over your diet. In some cases, hypothyroidism contributes to hypoglycemia and indirectly promotes weight gain. Timing meals and exercise to take advantage of the body's daily natural metabolic rhythms—combined with appropriate doses of T4 and T3—improves the odds of weight loss. Readers will learn a metabolism-enhancing weight-loss program, which includes a weeklong meal plan with low-fat, thyroid-friendly foods (yes, there are some foods that you should avoid!).

In general, a good diet is all that is needed to provide adequate nutritional support for people with hypothyroidism. But people with hypothyroidism may consider taking certain supplements in conservative measure.

Holistic and alternative treatments that can help stabilize hormonal fluctuations, manage stress, and regulate mind-body imbalances include meditation, yoga, homeopathy, and body work (e.g., massage). Though not integral to my approach, I do support patients who feel better when they try safe alternative approaches.

There is no cure for hypothyroidism. Achieving a balance with hypothyroidism is a lifelong process, a process based on self-awareness and devotion to continuing health.

It is my hope that this book will cast a new, hopeful light on your condition, that it will expose obstacles in your path to health and reveal ways for you to reclaim a steady, healthy rhythm in your life—one that allows you to move easily and energetically in your ever-changing world. In the following chapters, I will show you how and why your body has lost its balance and give you specific and practical guidelines that have proved effective for thousands of my patients. I am not offering any absolute answers. Each of you is unique, with a unique rhythm all your own. I hope you will gain a renewed sensitivity to your body's unique symptoms and a vocabulary for speaking convincingly with your physician to get the help you need to live your life to its fullest.

Chapter 2

First Stop: Diagnosis

When I first came to Dr. Blanchard, I was afraid to tell him all my symptoms because I'm thinking to myself that he's going to say the same thing that all the other doctors said: "There's nothing wrong. Your TSH is normal. Maybe you need an antidepressant." But when he said he thought I had hypothyroidism, it was unbelievable. Just knowing there was a reason for my symptoms . . . he gave me my life back.

—Jenna, aged thirty-eight

The road to wellness for people with hypothyroidism is clouded at every turn. The symptoms come on slowly and insidiously, often starting with fatigue or depression. Over time, symptoms accrue. One day you wake up and realize that the bad days outnumber the good, and you schedule an appointment with your doctor.

This, unfortunately, is where most patients are first blindsided.

In today's pressured managed-care environment, doctors have little time to hear and synthesize the many nonspecific symptoms of hypothyroidism. They hear palpitations, and it sets off an alarm for further cardiac investigation. Vague complaints of depression bring on prescribed antidepressants. The predominant or most disquieting symptom gets the most attention—and guides the next step: a prescription, an antidepressant, a referral to a specialist.

Like a needle on a broken record, many patients get stuck in a frustrated repeat pattern. They go from doctor to doctor, test to test, seeking out a name to confirm the symptoms that plague them. At worst they are shamed into believing that their symptoms are all in their heads. I have seen thousands of patients at the end of the diagnostic line, so to speak. *Unless you lobby for further investigation, many doctors won't suspect hypothyroidism.*

If you think that you have hypothyroidism, I highly encourage you to gather as much evidence as possible (use the work sheet on pages 103–106) and bring it with you to your next doctor's visit.

THE TSH TURNING POINT

If your doctor believes that hypothyroidism may be the cause of your symptoms or any physical findings, he or she will perform a TSH test. This is the defining point in the lives of most people with hypothyroidism. Your treatment (or lack thereof) will be determined by the results of this test. This commonplace approach to diagnosis is what Dr. John Lowe, director of research at the Fibromyalgia Research Foundation and author of the book *The Metabolic Treatment of Fibromyalgia,* calls "the tyranny of the TSH test." The common game plan is to treat hypothyroidism only if blood levels fall above the normal range of TSH. A high TSH indicates low thyroid function, or hypothyroidism, and the higher the TSH, the more severe the hypothyroidism.

Briefly, the test values used to define hypothyroidism are defined below, on page 28.

Start with a Neck Check

For many people, a goiter—an enlarged thyroid characterized by a fleshy roll around the bottom of the neck—is the first sign that something's wrong. If you have symptoms of hypothyroidism, you might not have a goiter. And you might never even have a tangibly enlarged thyroid. If you went to your doctor, he or she would perform a simple examination to see whether your thyroid is slightly enlarged. You can also do this at home. If you detect any unusual lumps or bumps, schedule an appointment with your doctor right away.

You'll need a small hand mirror and a glass of water.

1. Hold the mirror so that you can see the area of your neck just below the Adam's apple and right above the collarbone. This is where your thyroid sits.
2. While keeping your eye on your thyroid in the mirror, tip your head back.
3. Take a sip of water and swallow.
4. Watch your neck carefully for any bulges, enlargement, protrusions, or unusual appearance when you swallow. (Don't confuse your Adam's apple with your thyroid gland. The thyroid gland is very close to your collarbone.)
5. Repeat several times.
6. Report unusual lumps to your doctor right away.

Test Name	Normal Values (μU/ml)	Hypothyroid (μU/ml)
TSH Thyroid-stimulating hormone	0.3 to 3.04*	Over 3.1†
Total T4 Thyroxine	4.5 to 12.5	Under 4.5 when TSH is higher than normal
Free T4 Free thyroxine (FT4)	0.7 to 2.0	Less than 0.7
T3 Serum triiodothyronine	80 to 220	Less than 80
Thyroid peroxidase antibody	Less than 35 U/l	More than 35
Thyroid-binding globulin	13 to 39 μU/ml Pregnant: 27 to 66 μU/ml	More than 39 (more than 66 in pregnant women)

*Until November 2002, doctors had relied on a normal TSH level ranging from 0.5 to 5.0 to diagnose and treat patients with a thyroid disorder who tested outside the boundaries of that range. As of January 2003, the AACE encourages doctors to consider treatment for patients who test outside the boundaries of a narrower margin based on a target TSH level of 0.3 to 3.04. AACE believes the new range will result in proper diagnosis for millions of Americans who suffer from a mild thyroid disorder but have gone untreated until now.

†There is controversy over the limits defining hypothyroidism. Some studies indicate that levels over 2.0 may be abnormal.

What the Other Tests Measure

In addition to T4, your doctor may measure anti–thyroid peroxidase antibody, or anti-TPO. Anti-TPO detects the presence of antibodies against a protein found in thyroid cells. These antibodies are not normally present, so a high value usually indicates autoimmune damage to the thyroid, seen in conditions like Hashimoto's thyroiditis and Graves' disease.

To get from the thyroid to their target organs and work their metabolic magic, thyroid hormones connect up to proteins in the blood. They become "protein-bound." While protein-bound, hormone is inactive. Free T4 is a measure of the amount of *active* T4 in the blood. Similarly, free T3 measures the amount of unbound T3 hormone.

Any factor that changes the amount of proteins in the body can affect the total amount of free, active T4 and T3 in the body. Estrogen is one culprit. It makes more protein available. This locks up more thyroid hormone, leaving less free and active. Other chemicals and factors have the opposite effect. They lower protein levels. This means that more T4 and T3 are free and active. Examples are testosterone, corticosteroids, severe illness, cirrhosis, and nephrotic syndrome.

Define "Normal"

Literally millions of patients suffering from symptoms that clearly spell out hypothyroidism are denied treatment because of TSH levels that are falsely in the normal range.

My case against diagnosis and treatment by the numbers gets stronger every day. Consider a young Washington, D.C., patient of mine. At age thirty-two, she was the picture of hypothyroidism, but her doctor insisted it was all in her head. Two years before seeing me, in August 1998, Lisa's symptoms came on quickly. Though she'd never been thin, she never had real problems with her weight either. In the space of two months, she gained twenty-five pounds without eating more or exercising less. By four months, she was up fifteen more pounds. "It was a downward spiral," she told me. She recalled noticing that her eyebrows and hair were thinning (a cardinal sign), itching skin, and mental fogginess. "I didn't want to get out of bed. I was weepy and mopey—there were times when I was considering suicide."

Her primary-care physician ran some tests, and all were normal. "The doctor pooh-poohed me and said I was depressed over the weight gain. She prescribed Prozac and upped my dose to the highest limit."

When Lisa went to her brother's wedding, her friends from high school could barely disguise their shock. She'd gained forty pounds in just nine months, and in spite of treatment she still felt depressed. It was at this family event that she heard about a great-aunt who had suffered from thyroid problems. This information about her family history was an important clue, because it motivated Lisa to explore thyroid disease as a possible source of her problems.

Back to her doctor, who performed a TSH test—also normal. "Then I got active and searched the Web. I discovered that doctors were beginning to question the laboratory values. But my doctor didn't buy it and wanted to switch my antidepressant."

In our intake session, I noticed immediately her thinning eyebrows and puffy eyelids. According to Lisa, "Dr. Blanchard spent lots of time going through my history and said—and this is the most amazing thing—'Here's a list of twelve symptoms of hypothyroidism. You have ten of them.' And he said, 'You have a real illness. It's not in your head,'" she recalls. "I'm usually so reserved a person, but I thought I would start crying with relief at being validated."

Until the availability of the TSH test, diagnosis of hypothyroidism was based on symptoms. When the first sensitive test came out in the 1970s, it was considered a landmark event. And the reference range for "normal" has been carved in stone in the minds of clinical authorities ever since.

Normal values vary from lab to lab. What is a normal TSH result? The answer varies depending on which laboratory tests your blood, because reference ranges for what's normal vary slightly from lab to lab. Clinicians and patients alike are warned to always check to find out what the specific normal range is for the test value at *their* lab.

Other valuable tests are not often performed. While some doctors actively seek out answers to the TPO antibody test for autoimmune conditions, most do not. Remember the case of Jackie in chapter 1, who only convinced her doctor to investigate autoantibodies by "proving" her hypothyroidism with a TSH of 6. What is the fate of other patients who have a "normal" TSH but high autoantibodies?

The clinical definition of normal values is in flux. Even the medical establishment cannot settle on a boundary between normal and abnormal TSH results. A series of studies over the past decade challenged the notion that normal TSH levels are between 0.4 and 6.0 μU/l.

Dr. A. P. Weetman, a professor of medicine, in an article titled "Fortnightly Review: Hypothyroidism: Screening and Subclinical Disease," which appeared in the April 19, 1997, issue of the *British Medical Journal*, called into question the lab standards that have excluded millions of hypothyroid patients over the years:

> ... even within the reference range of around 0.5–4.5 mU/l, a high thyroid stimulating hormone concentration (>2 mU/l) was associated with an increased risk of future hypothyroidism. The simplest explanation is that thyroid disease is so common that many people predisposed to thyroid failure are included in a laboratory's reference population. ...

In February 2000, the Colorado Thyroid Disease Prevalence Study estimated that as many as 13 million Americans had undiagnosed thyroid disease. In this study, investigators used the standard diagnostic criteria to define hypothyroidism—that the TSH had to exceed the lab's normal range.

Finally, as we saw in chapter 1, the American Association of

Clinical Endocrinologists, the governing body for board-certified endocrinologists nationwide, revised the definition of "normal" for the TSH twice within two years. With the latest revision in January 2003, up to 27 million people with hypothyroidism are undiagnosed.

TSH levels may not actually reflect hormonal activity. This is the crux of my issue with TSH tests. Several factors can falsely suppress TSH test results:

- The conversion of T4 to T3 in the pituitary and at the tissue level as seen in mild hypothyroidism (as described in the next chapter)
- Serious illness (nonthyroid illness), which can reduce the production of TSH
- Antidepressants (e.g., Prozac)
- Glucocorticoids (anti-inflammatory drugs)
- Anticonvulsants (drugs for epilepsy)
- Cholesterol-lowering drugs
- Caffeine, which may reduce TSH production

DIAGNOSIS BY TRIAL

Instead of basing diagnosis on a test result, I suggest basing it on the patients' reports and medical history. I can personally attest to the fact that there are thousands of people with "normal" thyroid test results who experience the classic symptoms of hypothyroidism and who prove it by their excellent response to appropriate thyroid therapy. These individuals have, in essence, redefined hypothyroidism. In my experience, the combination of symptoms and medical history is much more telling than the TSH test, or any other test alone.

My Two-Week Diagnostic Trial: The Most Effective Diagnostic Tool

When I am satisfied that my patient has enough in favor of hypothyroidism (symptoms, signs, history), I recommend a therapeutic trial of thyroid hormone. As you'll see on page 50 where I outline my approach, I start patients with a very low dose of T4 and ask them to monitor their reactions, keeping in close touch with me, for two weeks. I will also order a TSH and a T4 test.

Why a TSH test? There are two reasons. The pattern of test results helps me understand the underlying *pathology* (the cause on a cellular level), which in turn helps me determine the best treatment. In addition, I am looking for each individual patient's "personal best"—at which levels does he or she feel best? This baseline is a helpful guide in fine-tuning each patients therapy, though symptoms are still of more importance.

During this trial period, I watch closely not only for symptom reduction but for any signs of thyroid treatment overdose—palpitations, tremors, rapid heartbeat. This is a particularly tricky situation in patients who present with cardiac problems, as I describe on page 74.

My patients' response to this trial is the starting point for a treatment plan—a plan that takes into account symptoms, core problems with the thyroid and hormonal processes, and a patient's stage in life. For example, diagnostic considerations are different for a pregnant woman than they are for a sixty-year-old man. At every life stage, the metabolic rhythms change, and with these changes, different treatment needs emerge. In part II, we'll look specifically at the life-stage-driven factors that influence thyroid disease . . . and health.

Chapter 3

❖

Going Against the Tide:
The 2 Percent Solution

As you've probably guessed by now, I believe that most doctors know less than half the story about treating hypothyroidism. Just as there's single-mindedness about using the TSH test, there's a steadfast loyalty to synthetic thyroxine, or T4. Doctors are convinced that the problem with hypothyroidism is on the production end and that if T4 levels were ample, then T3 would follow by enzyme conversion. To put a new twist on a great old song: All you need is T4. This is true *in some people.* If you're not producing enough T4 from your thyroid but you have a healthy metabolic conversion of T4 to T3, there's no need to add any other supplements. However . . .

Over the years, I noticed how many patients came to me because of the failure of T4 to help. This led me on a clinical mission to find another option. After many years of evaluating patients with different treatment options, I began to see beautiful responses to T3 and T4 in physiologic doses—my 2 percent solution.

In this chapter, you'll learn the mechanics of hypothyroidism, the scientific foundation for your symptoms (some proven, some theoretical), and a rationale for my unorthodox treatment incorporating T3 and T4.

I've tried to make this technical information accessible to anyone who's interested in understanding hypothyroidism. By mastering these concepts, you can become an active partner in optimizing your health with a willing and knowledgeable physician and have the basic knowledge to identify a good doctor in the first place. We begin with the thyroid gland.

POWERFUL HORMONES COME IN SMALL PACKAGES

The thyroid gland occupies only a small parcel of physiologic real estate, but its influence extends to every micromillimeter of the body's vast territory. Measuring only two to four inches in diameter, the butterfly-shaped organ perched at the base of your neck pumps out hormones that affect the energy production of almost every cell, in every tissue, in every organ in your body. It controls metabolism—the rate at which cells convert nutrients and oxygen into energy. It regulates body temperature, affects body weight, muscle strength, energy level, fertility, and more. With such broad-ranging effects, it's no wonder that thyroid disease can cause such a vast variety of symptoms.

As discussed in chapter 1, the thyroid stores much of the body's supply of iodine and is famous for producing two hormones, known collectively as thyroid hormone. They are thyroxine (known as T4) and triiodothyroxine (T3). T4 is made from an amino acid (amino acids are the building blocks of protein) called tyrosine and four iodine molecules. T3 is made by the enzymatic cleavage (detaching) of one iodine atom from the T4 molecule.

Iodine is crucial to the formation of these hormones. Too

much or too little can cause thyroid dysfunction and lead to a goiter, a swelling in the area where your neck meets the collarbone. (Iodine imbalance is just one reason for thyroid dysfunction. We'll look at other causes and risk factors in chapter 6.) T4 is more plentiful, but T3 is much more biologically active than T4. Only about 25 percent of T3 is actually formed in the thyroid gland. The rest is converted from T4 in the pituitary, bloodstream, and tissues such as those in the liver and kidney. The conversion is aided by a group of enzymes called deiodinase enzymes.

Once these thyroid hormones are in circulation, a large fraction attaches to other substances called thyroid hormone transport proteins, such as thyroglobulin, and it becomes inactive. In fact, only 0.03 percent of T4 and 0.5 percent of T3 are free and biologically active. But in the healthy individual, that's enough to keep the body's metabolic rhythm steady. Transporting proteins serve as storage bins for thyroid hormones, releasing them when the demand occurs.

The carrier proteins are important to the life span and potency of thyroid hormones. Their presence allows larger quantities of hormones to be ferried into the blood and delays their destruction. It is also thought that they play an important role in the availability of hormones to the placenta—the nutrient-rich environment for embryonic development.

In addition, the thyroid manufactures other thyroid hormones, including several types of T1 and T2, and reverse T3. According to conventional doctrine, these hormones are inactive and serve no purpose. I believe, as I will discuss below, that other products of the thyroid besides T3 and T4 are critically important to the body's health.

Supply and Demand

Conventional medicine confirms that the thyroid operates on a somewhat convoluted form of supply and demand. Hypothyroidism sets in when there is either a glitch in the supply end (from thyroid gland or the availability of hormones en route to tissues) or an unexpected increase in demand (stress, cold weather, weight gain, etc.—see chapter 5).

The pituitary and hypothalamus are middlemen in the manufacture and delivery of thyroid hormone. And the deiodinase enzymes make sure that thyroid by-products such as T3, T2s, and T1s are ample in supply.

The process begins when the hypothalamus detects a need for more thyroid hormone. The hypothalamus is located near the base of your brain. It is on the lookout for factors such as cold, heat, and stress that might influence the body's needs for energy and a variety of other hormone-mediated factors. It also scouts the bloodstream for thyroid hormone.

When the hypothalamus senses the need for more thyroid hormone, it calls out to the pituitary—via thyrotropin-releasing hormone (TRH)—to make a hormone known as thyrotropin, also called thyroid-stimulating hormone (TSH). Like the hypothalamus, your pituitary gland can scan the body and release a certain amount of TSH, depending on how much thyroid hormone is in your blood. Your thyroid gland, in turn, adjusts its production of hormones based on the amount of TSH it receives from the pituitary gland.

When the thyroid gland doesn't make enough hormones, the result is hypothyroidism. There are a multitude of conditions and risk factors that contribute to thyroid gland problems, which we'll explore in chapter 6. Depending on your age, your physiology, and your sensitivities, you then experience a cluster of symptoms, ranging from fatigue, depression, dry skin, and cold sensitivity to symptoms that masquerade as PMS, fibromyalgia, hypoglycemia, and irritable bowel syndrome (IBS), to name a few.

Here, in brief, is how conventional doctors view the interplay of hormones in hypothyroidism:

Hypothalamus detects need for increased T4 and T3 in the bloodstream and sends thyrotropin-releasing hormone (TRH) to pituitary

↓

Pituitary produces thyroid-stimulating hormone (TSH)

↓

Thyroid gland produces, stores, and releases more T4 and T3

↓

Deiodinase enzymes convert T4 to T3

↓

TSH test detects excess TSH levels, indicative of lower-than-normal T4 and T3 levels

↓

Treatment of patients is based on higher-than-normal TSH levels

But let's not sum up the problem so quickly—much more is happening here than is taught in medical school. Lots of things can happen to thyroid hormone to keep it from reaching its final destination besides inadequate production due to gland disease.

A main problem arises in the conversion of T4 to T3 and other "inactive" thyroid hormones. Why is this so important? Conventional doctors will tell you that only T4 is important (as evidenced by the fact that they only prescribe T4) because it eventually converts to T3 on its own—enough to satisfy our metabolic needs. So it is very important that T4 be converted to T3, even from the viewpoint of my more doctrinaire colleagues.

I am not alone in believing that T3 and the other allegedly inactive hormones play a critical role in our metabolic health. Before looking at how the conversion process can go wrong, let's examine the evidence supporting the use of T3 and other thyroid hormones.

The Hypothyroid Body Needs More Than Most Doctors Think

It is my belief that the majority of people with hypothyroidism need more than T4 supplementation. They also need T3 (and quite possibly the other Ts supplied only by natural thyroid). And the body requires these two hormones in physiologic doses that address deficits both in the thyroid gland and at the tissue level.

Based on close observation of thousands of patients, through twenty-five years of fine-tuning their doses, I arrived at the 2 percent solution: a physiologic ratio of 98 percent T4 and 2 percent T3.

A Look at Dr. Blanchard's Prescription Pad

Here is a brief review of my most widely used therapeutic options, with some remarks about their use.

A Variety of Levothyroxine Options

Although all of the following drugs are "100% synthetic T4," they do vary slightly. Some have dyes that spur allergic reactions in my patients; others have additives that somehow impact their performance. Through my guided trial and error, most patients can find a form of levothyroxine that meets their needs. See the Resources section at the back of this book for contact and Web site information on specific drugs.

Unithroid (Jerome Stevens Pharmaceuticals and distributed by Watson)
Levoxyl (King Pharmaceuticals)
Levo-T (Mova)
Synthroid (Abbott Laboratories)
Levothroid (Forest Laboratories)

What You Should Know About Taking Levothyroxine

Your doctor may prescribe levothyroxine to be taken as a single dose, preferably on an empty stomach, one-half to one hour before meals. Levothyroxine absorption is increased on an empty stomach and decreased by food (especially fiber) and some drugs. Note: if you've always taken your medication with food (or in some other way) and you're satisfied with how you feel, don't change! Suddenly "correcting" your regimen would change the way your medication is absorbed, and possibly its effectiveness. So don't fix what ain't broke!

T3 Options

In the United States, the only brand of T3 available is Cytomel (King Pharmaceuticals). Because of its short activity in the body, I routinely have my compounding pharmacist produce time-released capsules of T3 (see "Compounding Defined" on pg 41). In addition, I've had him put T3 into transdermal creams for a few patients who appeared to have GI problems with capsules. (By avoiding metabolism in the liver, it might in theory work better, too.) But because creams are more expensive to produce and do not seem to work better, I rarely use this option anymore.

Liotrix is a synthetic drug combination of T4 and T3. Thyrolar (Forest Laboratories) is the only brand available in the United States.

Compounding Defined

In the context of the pharmacy, compounding means making by hand. An analogy is a dinner. You can either prepare it from scratch—cutting, mixing, and cooking all of the ingredients to create a dinner to your taste—or you can buy a packaged precooked TV dinner. Compounding can be as simple as putting an existing drug into a time-release capsule or as complex as grinding different pills to specific proportions, adding flavor, and ensuring that they work in a slow-release cream form.

Although the practice of custom-preparing medications dates back to the origins of pharmacy, compounding's presence throughout the pharmacy profession has changed over the years. In the 1930s and 1940s, approximately 60 percent of all medications were compounded. During the 1950s and 1960s, with the advent of manufacturing, compounding declined. The pharmacist's role as a preparer of medications changed to that of a dispenser of manufactured dosage forms. In the 1980s, and especially in the 1990s physicians and patients again realized the benefits of preparing customized medications to meet specific patient needs. Today an estimated 43,000 prescriptions are compounded daily, 1 percent of total prescriptions dispensed. Also known as problem solvers, today's compounding pharmacists are using modern technology and innovative compounding techniques to meet specific patient needs.

For example, a patient may be allergic to a preservative

---

or dye in a manufactured product that compounding pharmacists can prepare in a dye-free or preservative-free dosage form. Some patients have difficulty in swallowing a capsule and require a lozenge. Many pediatric patients are noncompliant because their medications are bitter, but become compliant when the medication is flavored to their liking.

In order to achieve my therapeutic goals, I have had to develop my own dosage forms, which would not have been possible without the aid of my expert compounding pharmacists. T3 is central to my treatment regimen, but in its natural form it does not last long in the body, so for the convenience of my patients, I have it prepared in time-release capsules so that patients can take it once a day, instead of three or four times daily.

States require that pharmacy schools, as part of their core curriculum, must instruct students on the compounding of pharmaceuticals. While all pharmacists receive training in compounding, not all of them are equipped or willing to compound. To find a compounding pharmacist in your area, your doctor could consult the International Academy of Compounding Pharmacists for a referral (see Resources at the back of this book).

The Great Value of Natural Thyroid Extract

Natural thyroid extract is made from the desiccated thyroid glands of pigs, which, by an accident of biology, happen to have a pretty close thyroid hormone profile to humans. (Pigs are not killed specifically for clinical use; the thyroids are obtained from pigs used for meat.)

Until about 1960, natural thyroid extract was the treatment

of choice for hypothyroidism. Then came the advent of synthetic levothyroxine. Today there's a revived interest in natural thyroid extract—under the name brand Armour—due to glowing reports from patients. Unlike its synthetic counterparts, natural thyroid extract contains the entire range of active and so-called inactive hormones: T4, T3, T2s, T1s.

I was not always a natural thyroid advocate. I did not believe that it conferred much benefit over synthetic hormone. But at the urging of some patients and reports in the literature, I began to prescribe natural thyroid extract to a few patients who were not responding optimally to synthetic hormones. In the beginning, I saw a transient (fleeting) effect whenever I gave patients a short trial of natural thyroid extract: They felt wonderful for two months and then resumed symptoms.

It was then that I began to question my assumptions—a practice that has served me and my patients well over the years! I modified the doses, and now natural desiccated thyroid plays an important role in my list of therapeutic options. Hormone extract is particularly helpful in patients who have little or no functioning thyroid and cannot produce the trace hormones—T1s, T2s, and reverse T3—on their own.

Today I have a compounding pharmacist weigh out natural thyroid extract and put it into time-release capsules. I always prescribe synthetic T4 to balance the ratio in order to achieve 98 percent T4 and 2 percent T3. This approach has worked beautifully for many of my patients, especially those few who had nagging failures with synthetic hormone.

I am hopeful that the clinical community is opening its eyes and mind to the value of T3 (still considered an "alternative" treatment) and will embrace natural thyroid extract as well. This may, in turn, lay the foundation for more rigorous large-scale clinical studies that are now sorely lacking.

THE CLINICAL FOCUS BEYOND T4

Subtle shifts are happening in the static landscape of hypothyroid treatment. There are several studies describing the critical roles of T3 and T2 in the body. T3, for example, is a key player in the fundamental biological process of protein synthesis. Protein synthesis is the construction of cells—the making of new cells, repairing damaged cells, etc. Proteins are the stuff of life. A recent study in the *British Medical Journal* confirms that the brain needs T3 for adequate mental functioning and that it has a special affinity for thyroid-direct forms (versus T4, or the T3 that's been derived from T4). An estimated 25 percent of cells, according to some sources, can only use gland-direct T3.

A recent article in the *New England Journal of Medicine* showed that T3 improved the "well-being" of depressed hypothyroid patients. This study is described in more detail in chapter 5. Furthermore, there are many animal studies that clarify how T3 and the other Ts work in the body.

Perhaps it was these studies that provoked a reversal in thinking about T3 by staunch T3 opponent Anthony Toft. In response to the *New England Journal of Medicine* study mentioned above, Dr. Toft, a prominent and controversial endocrinologist, wrote an editorial questioning the therapeutic value of prescribed T3. Then in April 2002 at the twenty-first Joint Meeting of the British Endocrine Societies, Dr. Toft not only recanted his anti-T3 position but pronounced T3 as a valuable adjunct to T4 treatment. This is a landmark step on the part of the endocrinology establishment. It certainly helps legitimize the practices of doctors like me who were once considered on the fringe but are on the way to being regarded as pioneers.

In spite of this growing consensus, governing authorities in the United States still stand by their protocol: T4 only.

BACK TO THE CELLS

Problems in Preproduction—the Pituitary

Problems with conversion of T4 to T3 and other hormones could have a dire effect on the availability of these hormones to the body and to its metabolic vitality. Here's a brief review of how conversion goes wrong—and why doctors are wrong to believe that replacing only T4 will do the job in supplying T3.

It is a medical fact that the pituitary gland contains an enzyme called deiodinase. This is the enzyme that converts T4 to T3 at the pituitary level to prepare it for its use in the body. Remember that although T3 is not as prevalent as T4, it's much more active.

In the early stages of hypothyroidism, and particularly in patients with PMS (see Chapter 10), the deiodinase enzyme becomes hyperactive. Remember that in hypothyroidism, T4 and T3 levels in the bloodstream are initially low and insufficient for normal metabolic activity around the body. We rely on the pituitary to sense this lack and get the thyroid to step up production. However, the hyperactive deiodinase converts too much T4 to T3 at the pituitary level. It never senses the deficiency. Flooded with the high-powered T3, the pituitary is blinded to thyroid levels where they really count—in the bloodstream and organ tissues—and fail to get the cogs moving for thyroid hormone production.

Early-Stage Hypothyroidism: Too Much Hormone at the Pituitary, Too Little Where It Counts

Deiodinase activity heightens in pituitary
↓
T3 levels at pituitary increase
↓
Pituitary flooded with T3;
does not "sense" need for TSH secretion
↓
TSH lab results normal
↓
T4 and T3 levels in blood and target organs
diminished
↓
Hypothyroidism

In order for thyroid hormone to be beneficial in this situation, there must be a physiologic balance between T4 and T3 *at the tissue level.*

Meanwhile, back in the laboratory, the pituitary senses an excess of thyroid hormone, so the TSH test again tells us that everything is normal. (Remember: Since hypothyroidism is defined by higher-than-normal TSH results, the "normal" TSH in this situation is actually falsely suppressed.) Without the thyroid being stimulated to crank out more hormones, tissues become depleted, and your symptoms persist in spite of a normal TSH.

Problems at the End User—Organ Tissues

Deceptive practices occur not only in the pituitary but also in outlying areas—organ tissues. Another deiodinase enzyme changes T4 to T3 in a variety of other organs, such as the liver, kidney, and muscle. These tissues store T4, where it is changed to T3 as needed. It is an amazing function of the human body to sense the need for change, and to produce it—all in the name of survival.

I believe that when faced with waning supplies of thyroid hormone in the bloodstream, the body compensates by stepping up the conversion of T4 to T3 at the tissue level—with the help of deiodinase enzyme. This makes sense when you think about it: Making more powerhouse T3 is the body's way of compensating for a lack of T4. Thus, T4 becomes somewhat depleted, but T3 is relatively normal, maintained by increased conversion.

The result is an imbalance of thyroid hormones that may ultimately cause or worsen hypothyroidism. Blood tests taken at this time would show a low to normal TSH, which is interpreted as euthyroidism (normal thyroid function) or even *hyper*thyroidism. Meanwhile, the body suffers because there isn't enough thyroid hormone to do the job.

Very rarely, patients have tissue-level resistance to thyroid hormone due to a mutation in the gene that controls a receptor for T3, rendering it unable to bind with the hormone. The genetic mutation has been identified in only three hundred families.

Other Factors That May Disrupt T4–T3 Conversion

There is growing scientific evidence that adrenal insufficiency can impair the conversion of T4 to T3. In addition, some reports indicate that caffeine may stimulate the deiodinase enzyme and reduce TSH production.

Further, the deiodinase enzymes contain selenium, a naturally occurring nutrient, as a key structural element. I believe that a selenium deficiency can contribute to hypothyroidism. Selenium deficits may occur in people who consume vegetarian diets or who eat foods grown in selenium-poor soil. But too much selenium causes another set of problems. We'll discuss selenium and the value of supplementation in chapter 18.

Some researchers believe that self-produced antibodies to thyroid hormone (autoantibodies), as seen in people with Hashimoto's thyroiditis, can interfere with T4 conversion. This hypothesis is related somewhat to another, which posits that stress, which affects the immune system, may inhibit T3 conversion. These concepts have not yet been borne out in large-scale studies. However, they do provide a rationale for the central focus of my unique approach: the treatment of hypothyroidism symptoms in spite of normal TSH results, and the use of T3 or natural desiccated thyroid as part of the treatment protocol.

Chapter 4

— •◆• —

How I Work with My Patients:
Translating Theory into Practice

GETTING THE RATIO RIGHT—THAT IS,
PHYSIOLOGIC

The sixteenth-century physician Paracelsus said that any substance we put in the body is a poison until we find the right
dosage—then it's medicine. My treatment approach with the
physiologic 2 percent T3 is based on experience, confirmed by
my patients' almost universal success, and rooted in sound
clinical theory. In developing my approach, I intuitively followed my patients' responses as my guide to treatment. That
means speaking frequently with them, encouraging them to
talk to me and to tell me about even subtle shifts in how they
feel. This is why, over the years, I have never experienced serious adverse effects with T3. But I am very aware of potential
side effects such as heart palpitations and generally overstimu-
lated metabolism (hyperthyroidism). And, knowing that one

patient's salvation is another patient's poison, I make use of all therapeutic options available to me.

This chapter was written for two audiences: people with hypothyroidism and their caregivers. That includes clinicians. This chapter outlines all of the necessary steps to controlling hypothyroidism. Unfortunately, you cannot do it alone. You will need the help of an open-minded and caring doctor who is willing to take the steps needed to develop an individualized treatment plan that achieves the 2 percent T3 solution. It is a program of trial and error and fine-tuning. It involves interaction between physician and patient. It requires some patience. But the results, as thousands of my patients can attest, are life-affirming. Hypothyroidism robs people of their lives. My approach has given their lives back.

If your doctor is not willing to explore new strategies for treating hypothyroidism, seek out one who will. I refer you to chapter 19, "Finding a Doctor You Can Talk to—and Doing It Effectively," and to Mary J. Shomon's Web site for her listing of "top docs" across the country.

A STEP-BY-STEP GUIDE TO THE 2 PERCENT SOLUTION

The first step is to confirm suspicions of hypothyroidism. And the most conclusive way to confirm a diagnosis is through a diagnostic trial of thyroid hormone.

Step 1: My Two-Week Diagnostic Trial

When symptoms, history, and signs support a diagnosis of hypothyroidism, I confirm it with a short, closely monitored therapeutic trial. If you suspect you have hypothyroidism, but your doctor cannot confirm it through standard tests, share this information:

Patients not taking thyroid medication before:

- Start with 50 mcg (0.05 mg) of synthetic T4, taken in doses of one-half tablet daily. I usually give a sample package of seven pills.
- Monitor response. I ask patients to note changes in their energy levels, particularly late in the day. If they report late-day improvements within a few days of the trial, I tell them to call me. These patients have a very low-dose requirement, and they should not receive any higher dose.
- Identify underlying cellular problems. For example, patients who respond reasonably well to this regimen have highly active deiodinase enzymes. Their lab tests generally show T4 and TSH levels that are normal, but at the lower end.

In people already taking T4:

- If the TSH is 1 to 2 (normal), add T3 to get about a 98 percent T4 to 2 percent T3 ratio.
- If the T4 is high and the TSH is low and patients feel a little "hyper" (high pulse and rapid reflexes), reduce T4 before adding T3. T4 may need to be discontinued for a few days, since T4 effects dissipate slowly.
- If patients are undertreated, with a high or upper-range-normal TSH, introduce T3 and review in two to three weeks.

Step 2: Prescribe T3 and Monitor Response

- Adjust dosage to achieve physiologic T4:T3. After making an educated guess about T4 dosage, I have a time-release T3 capsule made up that will result in a 98 percent T4 to 2 percent T3 ratio. Your doctor will need to contact a compounding pharmacist (see Resources at the back of this book) to achieve this ratio.

- Add thyroid extract to existing T4 dose. Alternatively, I use natural extract with synthetic T4 (usually the dye-free 50 mcg tablets of Synthroid) to achieve the physiologic dose. If my patient is currently taking 100 mcg of T4, I add the smallest Armour pill (15 milligrams = ¼ grain) at one dose daily. With this dose I am adding only 9 mcg of T4 and 2.2 mcg of T3, thereby achieving the right 98:2 physiologic balance (about 109 mcg T4 to 2.2 mcg T3). The ultimate goal, as stated, is to achieve a physiologic dose that contains 98 percent T4 and 2 percent T3. Your physician will know that Armour contains a proportion that is too high: 80 percent T4 to 20 percent T3. To reach the right 2 percent solution, it is a matter of balancing with the right dosage of T4. The math is pretty straightforward.

  With their great response to this treatment, it might be tempting for some patients to want more Armour. Again, more is not better—even with natural thyroid extract.

- Return after three months for reevaluation. Patients will generally experience remarkable benefits over the first month or two, then feel their symptoms resume.

- If symptoms resume, increase T4 somewhat (full tablet on Mondays and Fridays; one-half tablet on other days). This reflects my repeated observation that adding physiologic doses of T3 slightly *increases* the need for T4 over time.

These *very general* guidelines provide a starting point for a lifetime of fine-tuning based on seasonal, life-stage, and other changes. In the more than twelve years that I have used this approach—prescribing T4 in spite of a normal TSH and adding T3 and/or natural extract to physiologic proportion—the worst effect has been a day or two of feeling "racy" palpitations, which were resolved immediately upon reduction of dosage. On the rare occasion that they occurred, these palpitations never progressed to serious cardiac problems.

Step 3: Individualize Treatment to Seasonal and Life-Stage Changes

No two patients are alike—and no two protocols are identical. Each individual presents his or her own unique therapeutic challenges and triumphs. These generalized recommendations can be applied and adjusted to keep pace with the changes in my patients' lives that occur from birth to old age.

- Thyroid insufficiency must be detected and corrected in pregnant women to prevent long-term cognitive (mental/learning) problems in children (chapter 8).
- Pregnancy can set off a lifetime of hypothyroidism for women; about 5 percent of pregnant women develop postpartum thyroiditis (chapter 8).
- Hypothyroid women do not have adequate thyroid reserves to carry a pregnancy, especially during the high-demand winter months, which helps explain the high rate of miscarriage in the late fall and early winter (chapter 8).
- Women diagnosed with hypothyroidism in their thirties and forties often trace their symptoms of PMS and depression to their teenage years (chapter 10).

- Men who experience loss of libido dovetailed with depression and social anxiety will see how my protocol helps address the underlying causes (chapter 11).
- Patients who report menopausal symptoms often benefit from addition of T3 or thyroid extract for their T4 treatment (chapter 12).
- Cardiac problems in advanced age could be an urgent sign of hypothyroidism, which increases dramatically with age (chapter 13).

In addition, as we'll see in the next chapter, specific clusters of symptoms, such as those suggesting fibromyalgia, depression, or irritable bowel syndrome, also present unique diagnostic and treatment challenges that can be overcome with my protocol.

BEWARE OF DRUG INTERACTIONS

The following drugs have been shown to interfere with thyroid hormone activity. Your doctor should be aware of all medications, both prescription and over-the-counter, that you are taking.

- Oral anticoagulants. Thyroid hormones can alter the activity of oral anticoagulants. Patients stabilized on oral anticoagulants who are found to require thyroid replacement therapy should be watched very closely when the treatment is started. No special precautions appear to be necessary when oral anticoagulant therapy is begun in a patient already stabilized on maintenance thyroid replacement therapy.
- Insulin or oral hypoglycemics. Thyroid hormone can increase the need for insulin or oral hypoglycemic agents. Patients receiving these drugs should be closely watched.

- Estrogen, oral contraceptives. Estrogens tend to increase serum thyroxine-binding globulin. In a patient with a nonfunctioning thyroid gland taking thyroid hormone, free levels will be decreased when estrogens are given. However, if your thyroid is secreting hormone, the decreased free thyroxine will be compensated by a higher hormone output by the thyroid.

- Tricyclic antidepressants. Use of thyroid hormone with imipramine and other tricyclic antidepressants may augment the antidepressant activity; fleeting cardiac arrhythmias have been observed. Thyroid hormone activity may also be enhanced.

- Digitalis. Thyroid hormone increases metabolic rate, which requires an increase in digitalis dosage.

- Cholesterol-lowering drugs. Cholestyramine and colestipol reduce the absorption of T4. These important agents can still be used if they are taken several hours before or after thyroid.

- Antacids. Carafate and aluminum-containing antacids may bind thyroid hormone in the gastrointestinal tract and reduce its absorption.

- Iron tablets or iron-containing vitamins (common over-the-counter medications) can interfere with hormone absorption. I always tell patients to take thyroid in the morning and iron with the evening meal.

DR. BLANCHARD ANSWERS QUESTIONS ABOUT TREATMENT

What's the best time of day to take thyroid hormone?

The manufacturers recommend that you take thyroid on an empty stomach, at least a half hour before eating any food. My recommendation for practical reasons is to set up a routine for taking thyroid that will be *convenient* and *automatic*. If you eat ten to fifteen minutes after taking thyroid pills, you'll probably need a higher dose. Since I would be judging your dosage based on your clinical response and changes in blood levels, it all evens out in the end as long as you stick with the same routine.

If you're splitting your daily dose of T3, then make sure that your second dose is well before your next meal.

Talk with your doctor about your schedule and work with him/her to create a plan that's best for you.

Can I take thyroid hormone with vitamins?

Given the practical problems of more than once-daily dosing, I advise taking vitamins and other supplements (except iron) together at least two hours after your thyroid medicine. If something in the mix changes the absorption of thyroid hormone, the dose adjustment, which has to be done anyway, will usually compensate.

Adding calcium to the mix further complicates matters. You need to keep two hours between calcium and thyroid hormone. I often suggest that my patients take calcium with their iron dose.

After a week on my new medication, I still don't feel any better. What should I do?

By now, you should have had some sense of improvement. However, it may take time to balance hormone levels, so give it another week or two and consult your doctor about slightly increasing your dose, or if you are only taking T4, ask your doctor to also prescribe a small amount of T3 to achieve a physiologic dose of 98 percent T4 and 2 percent T3.

I've heard that long-term thyroid hormone causes osteoporosis. Should I worry?

These concerns are based on a small study conducted in the

late 1980s by enthusiastic users of the new TSH test that for
the first time allowed diagnosis of hyperthyroidism (i.e., a low
TSH). The investigators noted that in a small number of patients thyroid hormone reduced hipbone density but not spine
density. Several larger-scale studies failed to confirm this finding. The original study found reduced hipbone density in patients with low TSH. It is possible that chronic thyroid
overdose contributes to osteoporosis, but such an observation
would be irrelevant, since overdose does *not* give patients additional benefit.

Since osteoporosis and the use of thyroid hormone are very
common, there are bound to be people who develop osteoporosis who are on thyroid hormone. It is my opinion that
proper doses of thyroid hormone will not cause osteoporosis,
and, in fact, thyroid hormone may help reduce the risk by increasing production of ovarian hormones and increasing the
energy to exercise.

**I'm feeling a little hollow and trembly on my new dose, but
my doctor says my TSH is normal. What's going on?**

If you're taking T4, you probably need a dose reduction.
You should let your doctor know if you feel in any way
hyper—fast or irregular heartbeat, shortness of breath, irritability, change in appetite, weight change, sweating, heat intolerance.

**I'm dragging! I live in Vermont, and I've been feeling pretty
good all summer with my dose of T4 and T3. But in mid-
September, I started feeling my symptoms come back. Help?**

Most patients who live in areas with big temperature
changes will begin to flag in the fall. Autumn often calls for an
increase in dose, with a corresponding reduction in the spring.
However, TSH levels fall in colder weather for patients on the
same dose of T4 year-round, so the physician will not have a

rising TSH to signal the need for more. In fact, the physician who slavishly adjusts according to minor changes in TSH will almost always adjust the dose in exactly the opposite way—i.e., *reduce* the dose in the fall/winter, because of a lower TSH—and vice versa.

For instance, if my patient is taking 50 mcg (0.05 mg) T4 once a day, I might suggest she double her dose for three or four days, then make it a once-daily dose with a double dose on Mondays. T4 takes time to work its way through the system. By "overdosing" for a few days, I am often able to achieve a faster balance, at a higher level, and patients feel better faster. In the spring, the corresponding adjustment would be to stop T4 completely for three or four days and then pick it up at six tablets per week.

I'm taking T3 time-release and I'm not feeling so great. Shouldn't I take more?

Just because *some* hormone is good does not mean that more is better—especially in the case of thyroid hormone. Here's why:

T4 and especially T3 are important variables in body metabolism. There is an optimum level for each patient, and patients can be overdosed and observe such symptoms as fatigue and weight gain reminiscent of how they felt when they were low. You cannot be sure on the basis of symptoms alone whether you are too low or too high. Of course, rapid heartbeat and tremor, for example, are telling symptoms of overdose. Yet it amazes me how often patients who feel they need more are actually overdosed. They are often amazed as well by the improvement that occurs when treatment is stopped for a few days and then reinstated at a lower dose.

I think I'm allergic to thyroid medicines because every time I take them I break out in a rash. What can I do?

Many patients with hypothyroidism, especially with an autoimmune component (Hashimoto's), have allergies and other immune problems. I have seen this over and over in my practice. You are not allergic to the T4 or T3 themselves, but to the excipients (binders, fillers, and other additives in drugs) or the dyes present in all the commercial pills, except for the 0.05 mg (50 mcg) size. Allergy can occur to thyroid extract because it is a crude mixture of many components of animal (pig) origin.

Are the T4 pills you're taking tinted? Almost all the commercial T4 tablets contain dyes that may cause allergic reactions, although the 50-mcg dose of all four major brands is dye-free. If my patients experience allergic symptoms, usually nasal irritation and congestion, I prescribe the 50-mcg dye-free pills. However, this can mean taking twenty to thirty pills a week—a lot of pills! With this many pills, you're exposed to more excipients, and different types of reactions emerge in some patients—pain, stiffness, and tenderness in certain "tender points" behind the neck and knees.

My solution is to have my compounding pharmacist use dye-free gelatin capsules and obtain pure crystalline T4 and T3 from the manufacturer. The idea for using pure hormone came after I had seen a high rate of headaches in patients taking Cytomel tablets. Compounding T4 and T3 in the same capsule without excipients often works well in patients with asthma or allergy symptoms. It may be pricier, but the dramatic improvement is often worth it.

I was taking Armour, and it wasn't working. So I went to a new doctor who put me on 100 percent T4. And I felt much worse! So we went back to Armour. Now I feel like I'm overdosing. What's up?

It's true that doctors who treat by the book will often take their patients off Armour and prescribe 100 percent T4, which produces an imbalance of T4 and T3 at the tissue level and will most likely cause greater symptoms. If a doctor prescribes 1 grain of Armour, he/she is adding 9 mcg of the much more powerful T3. The prior treatment with 100 percent T4 raised your tissue T4 levels much higher than they were before you started taking Armour (80 percent T4 and 20 percent T2). Thus, the amount of T3 that you tolerated before can now cause clinical symptoms of hyperthyroidism.

Chapter 5

———— •◆• ————

The Tale of the Mouse and the Lizard and Other Explanations for Your Symptoms

Now that you know more about hypothyroidism on a cellular level, let's look at how it translates into symptoms and how my treatment approach can help you to keep thyroid levels balanced and symptoms at bay.

WHY YOU FEEL COLD

Once, a mouse and a lizard were in a chilly storeroom looking for food. Night fell and the temperature dropped. The lizard's skin and entire body became very, very cold. In fact, he was almost exactly the same temperature as the surrounding air. Since he had no way of raising his own temperature to a healthy level, the lizard gathered as much energy as he could muster and climbed out the vent toward the heating unit. The mouse, being a warm-blooded vertebrate (i.e., a mammal), could survive in the cold because his body was hard at work, thanks to an internal process called thermogenesis. This basically means that like humans, mice generate ("genesis") their own heat ("thermo") in order to adapt to the cold. But thermogenesis isn't an isolated event like flipping a heat switch.

Interestingly enough, comparison of hypothyroid and normal animal muscle shows that, for any given amount of mechanical work, the normal muscle generates more heat. What this suggests is that the hypothyroid cell is less efficient in using energy and turning nutrients into heat than the normal muscle. As a result, if you have lower-than-normal levels of thyroid hormone in your body, you'll be less able to maintain a comfortable temperature, and your muscles may feel weak and prone to cramps.

OTHER MUSCULAR SYMPTOMS: FIBROMYALGIA

Muscle pain and tenderness (myalgia), joint pain (arthralgia), and joint swelling (effusion), along with sleep disturbances and debilitating fatigue, are the classic symptoms of fibromyalgia. They are also typical of hypothyroidism. In fact, while attending a lecture on fibromyalgia, I was struck by the thought that the symptoms displayed on the speaker's slides reflected hypothyroidism with a musculoskeletal focus. Like hypothyroidism, fibromyalgia is linked with autoimmune diseases. And like hypothyroidism, it is most common among women (nine out of ten sufferers are women).

One of my patients, Penelope, aged fifty-four, had suffered symptoms of hypothyroidism since she was a child. At our input session, she recalled always being cold and turning blue in the pool. Over the years, she developed small pains that in turn developed slowly into disability. A creative person, successful inventor, and consultant, Penelope had a very full career. But as the symptoms of fibromyalgia took hold, her abilities waned. In her words:

> I couldn't use a computer without being in pain. My assistant measured my decline in Post-it notes: I went from having more than 250 Post-its on my bulletin board to 100 to 50. People in walkers swanned past me in the park. I used to walk miles in New York City, and I couldn't walk a block without a two-hour nap. I lived on soup delivered from *downstairs,* and the delivery boy had to open the lid for me! I was at a mind-boggling pain scale: I was between 8.5 and 9 on the pain scale. I weighed 203 pounds, and I was at the end of my rope.

These extreme-sounding symptoms are, unfortunately, commonplace among people with fibromyalgia. Like many patients, Penelope had shuffled from doctor to doctor before landing in my office. Other doctors had labeled her hysterical, depressive, menopausal, and lazy. She was menopausal, but she was far from hysterical, depressed, or lazy. She was very rational, very well read about hypothyroidism and fibromyalgia, and I learned that in spite of her pain, she worked forty-plus hours a week. I could only imagine her capacity if she were well.

This patient had been taking Synthroid with 25 mcg Cytomel daily. She was also taking hormone replacement therapy, including estradiol and progesterone. Supplements included Ambien and kava for sleep. At the time of her initial visit, she had a very distorted thyroid profile: Her T4 was 3.8 (way below normal), and her TSH was 0.53 (near hyperthyroid). This profile is typical of patients taking too much T3.

I switched her to a lower dose of T3 and slowly changed her T3 and T4 doses until she was taking a physiologic balance of both (at the time, I was not using natural thyroid extract). This combination had a dramatically positive effect. On her own, Penelope supplemented this treatment with vitamin C, vitamin B_{12}, and SAMe, a nutritional supplement. Within three months, Penelope greeted me in my office at the end of a three-city business trip, with her carry-on luggage in tow—an impossibility before. Today, with the help of treatment and exercise, she has lost much weight and is proud to say that she wears skirts with thin pleats!

Penelope's experience is one of my best cases of fibromyalgia. I have honestly not enjoyed this level of success with other patients, though all of them experience some level of relief. This suggests that hypothyroidism may not be the only mechanism at work in fibromyalgia.

There are several theories about the origins of fibromyalgia that I consider useful, though I'm not convinced that anyone has come up with a satisfying answer. Probably the most accepted theory is that fibromyalgia is caused by sleep disturbances. This fits with the reports from my patients of fitful sleeping and frequent awakening, with drowsiness during the day.

A very interesting recent study also links sleep disturbances with weight gain and correlates the two problems with metabolic dysfunctions that occur with sleep deprivation. According to the 2002 study, published in both the *Journal of the American Medical Association* and the *Lancet,* sleep loss may increase hunger and affect the body's metabolism, which may make it more difficult to maintain or lose weight.

Specifically, sleep loss has been shown to affect the secretion of cortisol, a hormone that regulates appetite. As a result, individuals who lose sleep may continue to feel hungry despite adequate food intake. Additionally, sleep loss may interfere with the body's ability to metabolize carbohydrates and cause high blood levels of glucose, a basic sugar. Excess glucose promotes the overproduction of insulin, which can promote the storage of body fat, and can also lead to insulin resistance, a critical feature of adult-onset diabetes.

Though the researchers don't mention it, hypothyroidism is an invisible link to all of these conditions. It is associated with growth hormone disturbances, sleep disturbances, chronic fatigue syndrome, and insulin dysregulation. (More about this study in chapter 15.)

Another theory harkens back to the concept that patients suffer a defect in energy generation at the cellular level. This theory helps explain the fatigue, stiffness, and exercise intolerance. In a different study, the authors hypothesize that a deficiency in magnesium and malic acid (a compound found in apples) may be the source of the problem. Though some patients have responded to supplements of magnesium and malic acid, others have not.

This same mechanism—defect in energy production—is attributed to chronic fatigue syndrome (CFS). Indeed, there appears to be a connection between CFS and hypothyroidism. And there is evidence that individuals with chronic fatigue and/or fibromyalgia have difficulty in converting T4 to T3. Measurement of blood levels can miss this problem.

In addition, research by John Lowe, D.C., who specializes in fibromyalgia and thyroid disease, proposes that thyroid receptor resistance occurs in fibromyalgia. Some patients who fail regular thyroid hormone treatment respond dramatically to high-dose sustained-release T3 (though this was certainly not the case with my patient Penelope). Remember that everyone is unique and will respond differently to treatment.

Symptoms of Fibromyalgia and Chronic Fatigue Syndrome

- Pain lasting more than six months that affects your upper and lower body and right and left side with no known cause, like an accident (fibromyalgia)
- Brain fog for over six months that is not relieved by rest and that limits physical activity (chronic fatigue syndrome)
- Frequent infections such as chronic sinus inflammation/infection (sinusitis) and/or chemical/medication sensitivities
- Sleep disturbances for six months or longer that do not improve with rest and that limit your way of life
- Feeling worse or having greatly diminished energy and strength the day after exercise
- Bowel dysfunction. Many people diagnosed with irritable bowel syndrome (IBS) or spastic colon have chronic fatigue or fibromyalgia.

R. Paul St. Amand, M.D., author of *What Your Doctor May Not Tell You About Fibromyalgia,* put forth the concept that too much phosphate in muscle cells damages the muscle's ability to generate energy—again, similar to the study described above. St. Amand has championed phosphate depletion through the use of the medication guaifenesin as effective. While some other physicians and many fibromyalgia sufferers have received results through this protocol, other physicians have not.

Thyroid replacement with time-release T3 is very successful in my practice in eliminating symptoms of jerking or jumping muscles ("restless leg"), and sleep quality can be dramatically improved. Others have found tricyclic antidepressants to be somewhat effective in correcting the sleep disturbances typical of fibromyalgia. As with all patients, those suffering from fibromyalgia require individualized treatment, and I encourage them to try safe supplements and to find the mix that works best for them. In one small study, monosodium glutamate (MSG) was found to be the culprit: Eliminating this food additive resulted in a complete relief of symptoms. MSG is commonly used in restaurants and packaged foods to enhance flavor.

DEPRESSION AND SEASONAL AFFECTIVE DISORDER

The link between depression and hypothyroidism is strong. The Thyroid Society estimates that up to 15 percent of people with depression also have hypothyroidism. And often it becomes worse with seasonal changes. Over the years, I've noticed that my patients can hum along for months in the summer on a certain dose, and as autumn approaches, they start to flag.

It is my belief that seasonal changes to colder temperatures draw on thyroid reserves and can cause or worsen symptoms of hypothyroidism, not only creating cold intolerance but also bringing about depression/seasonal affective disorder (SAD), joint stiffness, dry skin, and a host of other hypothyroid symptoms that could easily be passed off as winter ailments.

One of my patients, Robert, had some improvement with T4 prescribed by another physician until the cold weather set in. In his words:

I had a VP position at a major health care company. I'd put on weight. I was falling asleep at the office and praying that no one would walk in when I closed my eyes. One day I even fell asleep on a conference call. No amount of conditioner could help my hair, which was so brittle. Luckily, I found a D.O. [doctor of osteopathy] who did a full workup. He came back and said my TSH was 11—I had no functioning thyroid. The biggest issue was depression. I'd always been this outgoing energetic funny guy. And I didn't recognize that I became completely antisocial. The D.O. put me on Synthroid, and in two weeks I'd say I felt 20 percent better, but then I plateaued and I was right in the normal range with the blood test. For the next few years, even with the Synthroid, I just felt really lousy during fall and winter.

Then I moved to Boston, and I saw Dr. Blanchard's name on Mary Shomon's Web site. I started seeing him during the winter months. He just looks at me and knows, and he asks me all the questions I was afraid to ask other doctors, or I thought if I asked they'd think I was losing my mind.

With confidence he said, this time next year you'll feel much better.

Increasing Robert's T4 and T3 doses about 20 percent during the winter months dramatically improved his symptoms. Like most of my patients, he is on a seasonal schedule, returning each spring and winter for his seasonal dose adjustment.

My standard practice of reevaluating patients during times of abrupt seasonal change is based on experience, not clinical studies. Most doctors would dismiss this approach. But when you see it again and again, and see virtually *all* patients feel substantially better after two to three weeks of appropriate adjustments, you know that it is the right way to go.

A recent report from the South Pole gives interesting insight into seasonal hypothyroidism. The study strongly suggests a link between reduced levels of T3 and SAD.

SAD is characterized by depression, poor concentration, irritability, and impaired memory during the winter months. In the Antarctic, it appears that people suffer from an especially debilitating form of SAD—known as polar T3 syndrome. Other symptoms include a striking reduction in physical strength and endurance. People suffering from this disorder also have below-normal body temperatures, and their energy requirements rise by as much as 40 percent, so they typically feel cold and eat more than usual.

Sound chillingly familiar?

The scientists in the South Pole study compared the effects of thyroid supplementation to those of a placebo (an inactive substance) in people who were diagnosed with polar T3 syndrome. The study confirmed that extended winter conditions reduced circulating thyroid hormone levels. Thyroid supplementation helped improve mood and mental skills, but it did not help much with exercise performance or body temperature. Perhaps this is due to the inefficient muscular use of thyroid hormone in hypothyroid patients. It is also possible that the brain is in more dire need of thyroid than muscles, and grabs the supplemental T3 first. I suspect that the dosage used was too low (as I've seen in my seasonal upward adjustments of thyroid replacement).

The fact that this study was conducted in people without confirmed hypothyroidism makes the results all the more dramatic for patients who live in more temperate regions. Because individuals with preexisting hypothyroidism already have depleted thyroid reserves, it doesn't take an arctic wind to induce symptoms. I have seen the same syndrome in thousands of patients who live in the comparatively tropical climate of Boston. More important, I have observed gratifying symptom reductions with seasonal dosage adjustments.

More on Depression

I think I was depressed as a child, tired and lethargic, and during adolescence. We didn't really talk about being depressed, so I struggled with it for a long time. I eventually went to see someone, and they put me on antidepressants, but I had a terrible reaction to them. It seemed like each cycle was getting worse, every month. I was suicidal. It was awful. I was ready to be committed. When I came to Dr. Blanchard and he told me there was something *physically* wrong with me, I cried. It was something legitimately wrong. I was crazy but I wasn't crazy! I'm able to focus now. I still get down and depressed, but it's manageable. I changed jobs, I got a really good job. I just wish that Dr. Blanchard had been around sooner. The last twelve years have been great.

—Risa, age fifty-five

It makes me sad to realize how many people there are out there who never find fulfillment in their work, whose marital relations break up—there's no purchase on life, so to speak. Many times when they come to me, they are taking six different drugs for psychiatric symptoms. The drugs have adverse effects, so they've been given another drug to counteract these side effects. By the time they reach my office, I have to unravel a knot of symptoms and treatments.

My first instinct is to remove the antidepressants in order to perform a clean trial of hormone replacement. But of course one worries that this could set off a serious depressive episode. Yet the antidepressants are causing their own problems such as weight gain and mental fogginess. It's a delicate balance.

THE FAT CONNECTION

Fats and thyroid hormone are critical cohorts in thermogenesis and metabolism in general. In their effort to control the body's thermostat, thyroid hormones help to metabolize fats (a.k.a. lipids).

If we could look into the cells of the cold mouse, we'd see T3 and T4 busy at work converting fat to energy (like stoking the metabolic fire). Fat cells are preoccupying way stations for thyroid hormone. The heavier you are, the more cells you have in your body. Although there may be technically enough thyroid hormone in the body to keep TSH levels normal, there might not be enough to do the rounds in the rest of the body. As a result, overall metabolism declines, and other body systems become sluggish. A vicious cycle sets in: The heavier you are, the more hormone you "consume," which depletes other tissues and leaves your hormone-deprived body cold, tired, and mentally foggy. Not exactly an inspiring starting point for an exercise regimen.

The bad news is that thyroid replacement is not a magic diet pill. You won't lose weight just by taking thyroid hormone. This was once thought to be true. But today we know that excessive amounts of T4 can cause cellular resistance, crippling your body's ability to make use of thyroid hormone.

The good news is that replacing missing thyroid hormone can level the playing field, giving you the energy and the metabolic base for weight loss (chapter 15). According to the 2002 study mentioned on page 64, getting a *good* night's sleep can also help keep your weight down by taking advantage of the body's natural metabolic rhythms.

Excess weight is not just an aesthetic anathema; it can be a dangerous health risk. It contributes to other metabolic disorders such as diabetes, and it stresses the heart. Studies show

---

Conventional thyroid treatment actually promotes weight gain. In many people (but not all), treatment with synthetic 100 percent T4 can produce excessive T4 levels (at the upper end of normal) and TSH levels near the bottom of normal, nudging at hyperthyroidism. This creates a situation by which individuals feel hungry (from the metabolic thrust) but very fatigued due to excessive T4 replenishment and decreased conversion to T3. They ask their physicians for more T4 to handle their symptoms, but are denied because of their near-toxic levels.

---

that thyroid levels and lipids are inversely related: that is, the higher the thyroid level, the lower the fat level. On the other hand, when thyroid hormones are in short supply, lipid levels rise. And most of us are well aware of the hazardous cardiac effects of high cholesterol and triglycerides. Hypothyroidism also contributes to higher levels of the amino acid homocysteine, another cardiac risk factor.

More on Fat: The Insulin-Thyroid Connection

Every cell in the body needs glucose (sugar) as a source of energy. Glucose, as you may know, is quickly converted to fat unless it is used up in the form of energy. Every holiday season is testimony to the fact that eating lots of sugary foods leads to weight gain—and new year's resolutions to exercise.

Here's what happens: After eating, blood levels of glucose rise. The pancreas responds by producing a hormone called insulin. Insulin essentially puts a cap on glucose production by helping cells to pull glucose from the blood for use as energy. If glucose levels drop too low, the pancreas stops producing insulin.

There is a known connection between diabetes, a dysfunction in insulin production, and hypothyroidism. Fifteen to 20 percent of people with type I diabetes (insulin-dependent), as well as their siblings and parents, are at a greater risk of testing positive for a thyroid disorder. And at least 10 percent of people with type I diabetes develop chronic thyroiditis (inflammation of the thyroid), which can become frank hypothyroidism. Conversely, I believe that hypothyroidism also contributes to glucose disorders. Hypothyroidism slows the pancreatic response, allowing a greater rise in glucose after a meal, followed by overproduction of insulin. When glucose becomes absorbed into cells and levels decline in the blood, hypothyroidism inhibits the pancreas from stopping insulin production. These dysfunctions lead to symptoms commonly called hypoglycemia.

While hypothyroidism isn't a simple direct cause of obesity, I do think that along with disordered glucose-insulin metabolism, it helps promote weight gain. Individual eating patterns may be significantly affected by the need to prevent hypoglycemia. In other words, to stave off hypoglycemia, you may eat more than you normally would. The probability for increased insulin production is much higher for people with this type of metabolic disturbance, leading to overproduction of insulin and building fat stores.

In my experience, the vast majority of hypothyroid patients with symptoms suggestive of hypoglycemia—hunger, tremors, dizziness, fatigue, etc.—improve greatly with my approach to thyroid hormone replacement.

GETTING TO THE HEART OF HYPOTHYROIDISM

The heart is highly sensitive to thyroid hormone. But doctors are much more attuned to heart problems than they are to hormonal ailments. A typical scenario is a young woman who complains of frequent palpitations. (Palpitation usually refers to rapid heartbeats that have not been triggered by emotional or physical stress.) The problem may be so severe that this otherwise healthy woman ends up in the emergency room, where she undergoes elaborate and expensive evaluations that reveal nothing. In some cases, a diagnosis of mitral valve prolapse (MVP) is given due to detection of "systolic click."

Several years ago I began to believe that in hypothyroidism, the deiodinase enzyme is stimulated at all body tissues, including the cardiac muscle cell, to convert T4 to T3. In its attempt to compensate for the overall depressive effects of hypothyroidism (and sluggish heartbeat), T3 conversion is stepped up at the cardiac tissue level.

Cardiac muscle cells have prominent receptor sites for the T3 hormone. In essence, one has "T3 hyperthyroidism" at the level of the cardiac muscle cell, while surrounding tissues are actually somewhat hypothyroid.

The hypothyroid heart masquerades as many cardiovascular problems:

- Arteriosclerosis. As mentioned, hypothyroidism can cause a leap in lipid levels. It can raise levels of homocysteine, a potent contributor to coronary disease. These changes can cause narrowed, hardened arteries, a forerunner of heart disease and stroke.
- High blood pressure. Thyroid depletion renders arteries stiffer and less flexible, increasing the pressure needed to circulate blood around the body. The problem is high sys-

tolic blood pressure, the top number of the blood pressure reading. A blood pressure of 120/80 is considered healthy.

- Reduced heart rate. The thyroid slows the body down in many ways, including the rate at which the heart beats. In the extreme, hypothyroidism can cause bradycardia, an unusually slow rate.
- Weaker pumping. All of the above factors conspire to inhibit the heart from pumping as forcefully as it should. This can reduce blood flow to the skin, kidneys, brain, and other vital tissues.

Hypothyroidism has an ill effect on the heart, regardless of its severity. The mild, persistent reductions in thyroid hormone typical of what is called subclinical hypothyroidism may also put patients at higher risk of serious cardiac problems, including early heart attack, though in the clinical literature, studies are conflicting. In subclinical hypothyroidism, these effects can be especially insidious, since patients do not even have hypothyroid symptoms, and heart risks are usually silent as well.

Cardiac problems are more likely to arise if you have other risk factors besides hypothyroidism. Unfortunately, some of these factors come part and parcel with hypothyroidism, such as excess weight and lack of exercise—another reason why it is so important to restore normal thyroid levels in your body. Some studies show that replacing the missing thyroid helps reverse hyperlipidemia (high fat levels).

THE BRAIN FOG MACHINE

Extensive research on the developing brain and nervous system has found that thyroid hormones help orchestrate the elaborate process that is required for normal brain development. These hormones stimulate the production of nerve cells and the connecting links (dendrites) between the cells. Many studies connect thyroid levels to the brain's cognitive ability to process thoughts and to reason. Science informs us, for example, that thyroid hormones help maintain brain cell life, whereas a lack of thyroid hormone shortens the life cycle of brain cells. Although there are few studies exploring this phenomenon, one can easily imagine how hypothyroidism could reduce memory and produce "brain fog."

In my experience, the mental fogginess and memory lapses experienced by hypothyroid patients are among the most difficult symptoms for them to cope with. Here are some of the vivid ways my patients describe the effects of thyroid depletion on their mental capacity:

> The brain fog was intense. I clearly remember once walking up the stairs at my house to go get something, and halfway up, I'd forget what I was going to do, then I'd think of something new I would do when I got up and I would forget the second thing I would do when I got to the top of the stairs. I'd forget the names of people I'd known for years, people I worked with every day. I'd lost my personality. I was always this outgoing, funny person. I had lost all of that.
>
> —James M., aged forty-three

> The most annoying thing about this disease is that it's like having wool between your ears, what I call fuzzy thinking: everything seems to work in slo-mo. I was a teacher, curriculum developer, and the life of the mind was important to me. It's a low-level mental cloudiness that is very annoying and sometimes outright depressing.
>
> —Rhonda, aged thirty-four

One of my most serious problems was the fog. I was just getting by. I had managed to graduate from business school with honors, and then I entered a program for the certified financial analyst program. The test is given over a period of three years consecutively, and I remembered I barely passed the Level 2 test. It was a grueling day—I think it's an eight-hour test. A year later after having seen Dr. Blanchard, it was just a different test. I passed with flying colors. I just knew it. I wasn't fatigued; I had all mental processes available to me.

—Belinda, aged forty-five

These patients improved dramatically with a combination therapy of T3 and T4 as hormone replacement. Though I've been administering T3 supplements for over ten years, it appears that studies are beginning to show that the brain is quite sensitive to the effects of this hormone, carving out a legitimate place in the conventional doctor's prescription cabinet.

A 1999 study in the *New England Journal of Medicine* made big news in the thyroid community. Throughout two study periods, the patients were tested for their cognitive, mood, and physical capacities. The point was to compare the effectiveness of the two regimens.

In one trial period, subjects were studied on their usual dose of T4. In the other period, 50 mcg of T4 was replaced by 12.5 mcg of T3. This was done because of an old teaching (wrong in my opinion) that each mcg of T3 is "bioequivalent" metabolically to 4 mcg of T4. Despite much literature to the contrary, I believe the dose of T3 was higher than optimal, so the benefits of T3 were actually underestimated in this study.

There were almost no differences between the regimens regarding physical effects. But mental functioning improved dramatically in the patients taking combination therapy. And in a questionnaire, 65 percent of patients preferred the combination therapy to their previous T4 treatment. Only two patients preferred T4.

In another well-regarded study, T3 was found to hasten the normally slow-acting effects of standard tricyclic antidepressant treatment. The addition of T3 to the regimen cut in half the time it took for the drug to take effect—from twenty-two to eleven days.

It is well established that brain development of the fetus and newborn is critically dependent on adequate levels of thyroid hormone. A recent, highly publicized study from the National Institutes of Health shows that hypothyroidism in the pregnant mother is linked to a somewhat lower IQ in children. These results make a strong case for monitoring the thyroid function of pregnant women, especially in the first two months of gestation, when brain development is occurring entirely in the thyroid environment provided by the mother.

In another study, children with congenital hypothyroidism aged seven to twelve scored lower than other children in visual/spatial abilities, attention and focus, and mathematic prowess. The earlier their thyroid levels were normalized, the better they performed. Indeed, learning disorders similar to attention deficit disorder (ADD) have been linked with hypothyroidism. Replacement therapy with thyroid hormone has proved vital in preventing these difficulties in newborns, and later in life. We'll look more closely at these and other studies in chapter 9.

STRESS AND THE ADRENAL LINK

The adrenal glands are manufacturing plants and storehouses for hormones that help you cope with immediate stress (adrenaline) and long-term stress (cortisol). For people with hypothyroidism, the adrenal glands also produce hormones that aid in the conversion of the plentiful T4 to the scarcer but more potent T3, and may even affect their entry to cells. So when there is a problem with the adrenal machinery, it may affect thyroid production and result in hypothyroidism.

Like the thyroid, the adrenals work with the hypothalamus and the pituitary to make cortisol and adrenaline. Adrenaline helps the body to cope with crisis situations. Imagine the way you feel when something frightens you. Your stomach tenses up, your muscles contract, your heart pounds, and your mouth becomes dry. These are real physiologic responses to stress, coined in the 1930s as the "fight or flight" response by Harvard physiologist Walter B. Cannon. This defensive mechanism serves an important immediate purpose: to flee in the face of wild animals (or oncoming traffic). Once the stress is removed, the body returns to normal, and adrenaline levels drop.

More chronic, ongoing stress summons the adrenals to pump out cortisol. Illness, injury, and severe emotional upset are examples of more severe chronic stressors. Cortisol helps the body bear up against the low-level stresses in life. The adrenal system can become dysfunctional when stress is unrelenting. Not just the response to acute stress like an oncoming truck, but the chronic stress of coping with the growing demands of an everyday life. This is a type of stress that our bodies were not built to take for too long. Then there's the baseline stress that healthy bodies should readily adapt to, the ones that are part of the fabric of everyday life: changes in temperature, menstruation, walking up a steep incline. And in the report mentioned earlier, inadequate sleep can also heighten cortisol levels. People with hypothyroidism have problems coping with the physiologic stresses, which cripples the body for coping with higher levels of stress.

Eventually, the very hormones that save it in a crisis can

cause the body's demise when released on an ongoing basis. Science has linked high cortisol levels with immune dysfunction and related illness, such as the inability to fight infection and, as posited in the excellent book by Ridha Arem M.D., *The Thyroid Solution,* thyroid conditions such as Graves' disease and Hashimoto's thyroiditis. Dr. Arem argues that with a dysfunctional immune system, the brain may mistake the thyroid for a virus or other threatening invader and erroneously launch an attack on the thyroid.

A recent study indicates that chronic fatigue syndrome (CFS) may be linked to subtle changes in the hormonal stress response system called the HPA axis, traceable to significantly lower response levels of adrenal hormone.

The adrenals also produce a hormone called DHEA (dehydroepiandrosterone). DHEA is the precursor to sex hormones such as estrogen and testosterone. (A precursor is a hormone that leads to the production of other hormones.) Interference with DHEA production can lead to impotence, fertility problems, exaggerated menopausal symptoms, PMS, and more—all characteristic of hypothyroidism (see chapters 8 and 12).

Cortisol levels may also rise when thyroid medication does its metabolic-boosting job. For this reason, if your symptoms are not relieved by individualized treatment of thyroid replacement, your doctor should investigate your adrenal function. Treatment of low adrenal function may be as simple as taking very small amounts of cortisol each day. Supplements that support the adrenal system can also help and will be reviewed in Chapter 18. Though I'll touch on it in the next chapter, I refer patients to Richard and Karilee Shames's fine book *Thyroid Power* for detailed instructions on coping with adrenal insufficiency. In addition to Mary J. Shomon's Web site www.thyroid-info.com, I also refer patients to Dr. Joseph Mercola's excellent Web site www.Mercola.com.

Here's a brief look at the mechanisms at play with other hypothyroid symptoms.

HAIR LOSS, SKIN DRYNESS, NAIL BRITTLENESS

The thyroid controls the functioning of the skin, hair, and nails. Grease glands (sebaceous glands that produce sebum) are also influenced by the thyroid. People with hypothyroidism experience hair loss and brittleness. Their skin becomes dry and possibly itchy, with thick patches (particularly on the heels and elbows). Nails turn brittle and break easily.) In short, the symptoms include:

- Absence of sweating
- Brittle thick nails
- Bruising
- Coarse, dry scalp and hair
- Hair loss of the scalp, groin, outer eyebrows, etc.
- Pale, cold, scaly, wrinkled skin
- Poor wound healing
- Edema (swelling of the hands, face, eyelids)
- Yellow/ivory skin color

When hair loss is noticeable (more hair in the hairbrush or bathroom drain) but there are no identifiable patches of baldness, hypothyroidism should be suspected as a cause.

Hair grows at a steady rate of about a half inch a month for up to three years, when it goes into a resting period. One in ten hairs is in a resting period at any given time, and every three months or so, a new hair drives the old one out. Hypothyroidism can slow down this process, causing more hairs to go into hibernation, so that reject hairs are not replaced as quickly as they could be. Since hair growth is comparatively low on the survival chain (in these modern times, anyway), hair loss may be one of the first things you notice. Your thyroid reserves are diverted to more important functions, such as heat production and brain function.

Similarly, skin cells turn over at a regular rate. The lack of blood circulation (which brings oxygen and nutrients to the skin) combined with a slower rate of cell turnover can contribute to pallor and dry skin. In addition, the skin may turn sallow and yellowish due to disruption of vitamin A metabolism.

Swelling of the skin around the eyes is another distinctive hypothyroid feature which is often accompanied by facial swelling.

LOW LIBIDO

Men and women alike complain that when their thyroid levels take a dive, so does their sex drive. I make light of this situation, but it can be a serious problem that compounds depression and adds to relationship difficulties. Both reduced and excess thyroid hormone can upset the balance between testosterone (male hormone responsible in large part for our sex drive) and estrogen (female sex hormone). Men may experience impaired sperm production and difficulties with erections.

People with Hashimoto's autoimmune thyroiditis may also be at risk for other autoimmune diseases such as Sjögren's syndrome, which is characterized by dry, gritty eyes. See chapters 6 and 7 for more details.

IMMUNE PROBLEMS

The immune system is vulnerable to hypothyroidism in two ways. First, like other body systems, the immune system is susceptible to the torpor-inducing effects of hypothyroidism. People with hypothyroidism seem to be more susceptible to colds and flu, which tend to linger longer as its indolent immune system struggles to rally its depressed forces. But there may also be another mechanism at work. As mentioned earlier, Hashimoto's thyroiditis is the most common type of hypothyroidism; it is caused by an autoimmune dysfunction.

With autoimmune thyroiditis, the body's immune system mistakenly attacks its own cells—in this case the thyroid. This is a big topic that we'll explore in chapter 6. But what's important to know now is that people with one type of immune disorder are at risk for others. It is possible, though not proved, that a generalized immune dysfunction that stymies the immune system's ability to fight infection may be related to the underlying problem of thyroid autoimmunity.

Allergy symptoms may also flare up when you have hypothyroidism—another sign of immune dysfunction. Except in this case, it is your body's hypersensitivity to outside invaders that causes your symptoms, which may include tearing of the eyes, rashes and hives, and gastrointestinal complaints.

GASTROINTESTINAL COMPLAINTS

Alternating bouts of painful constipation relieved by diarrhea (especially at the time of a woman's menstrual flow) with cramping, abdominal bloating, and weight gain characterize the most common diagnosis by gastroenterologists today: irritable bowel syndrome (IBS). It is a diagnosis that gastroenterologists almost universally fail to link with hypothyroidism.

I believe that in the menstruating woman, IBS is a manifestation of hypothyroidism acting on two body systems: the bowel wall and the hormonal system that regulates menstruation.

As with other parts of the body, depleted thyroid levels reduce the normal muscular activity of the bowel walls, causing constipation and abdominal muscle cramps. The cramps and bloating can be so severe that they send patients to the emergency room—and even the operating room for exploration.

In one recent study, a patient came to the doctor with severe abdominal pains and swelling (ascites) that were misdiagnosed as abdominal cancer. She showed some signs of hypothyroidism (gravelly voice, dry skin, general pallor, high systolic blood pressure). But what threw them off track was when they took measurements of a cancer marker in the blood called CA 125; the levels were extremely high—as high as those seen in people with ovarian cancer. It was not until they performed biopsies and imaging tests that indicated no tumors or masses that they suspected another mechanism at work. The hoarse voice and dry skin motivated the doctors to test the woman's TSH, which was sky-high, indicating severe hypothyroidism.

The diarrhea occurs around the time of the period because it is a part of the premenstrual syndrome. As we'll see in chapter 10, hypothyroidism heightens the symptoms of PMS. In PMS, there's a powerful hormonally influenced retention of fluid (bloating) that often results in weight gain, sometimes ten pounds or more. Events leading to menstrual flow release the fluid, and weight loss is rapid.

Both sides of IBS—cramping and constipation combined with PMS-like symptoms—have been successfully relieved with combined 98 percent T4 and 2 percent T3 treatment.

By now, I hope you are convinced that your symptoms are not in your head. And you're armed with information to convince doubting doctors the same!

HYPOTHYROIDISM SYMPTOMS AND THEIR MECHANISMS: A BRIEF OVERVIEW

Here's a summary of the symptoms and hypothyroidism mechanisms behind them that you can show to your doctor:

Check If You Have Symptom	Symptom	Hypothyroid Mechanism or Contributing Factor
	Cold intolerance	Autoimmune: Raynaud's syndrome. Sluggish conversion of nutrients and oxygen to heat.
	Muscle cramps and tenderness	Defect at cellular level in energy conversion. Autoimmune: link with fibromyalgia.
	Fibromyalgia Tired, aching muscles Exhaustion after exercise Sleep disturbances Restless leg syndrome	Difficulty in converting T4 to T3.
	Brain fog (forgetfulness, sluggish thinking, loss of energy for life)	Inadequate levels of thyroid in brain, particularly T3 due to lack of T4 conversion, or thyroid dysfunction.
	Depression	Same as brain fog, above.
	Seasonal (cold weather) exacerbation of symptoms	Increased demand on metabolism (e.g., cold weather) with little thyroid reserve results in symptoms.
	Weight gain	Reduced metabolism enlarges fat cells, which sequester T4, causing hormone depletion and further sluggishness. Disordered insulin metabolism (10 percent) of people with type I diabetes develop chronic thyroiditis and hypothyroidism). Hypothyroidism slows the pancreatic response.
	Hair loss (nonpatchy) Skin dryness Nail brittleness	Slowing down of process of cell turnover and tissue/hair production.

Check If You Have Symptom	Symptom	Hypothyroid Mechanism or Contributing Factor
	Low libido	Low thyroid levels disrupt the balance of testosterone and estrogen.
	Infertility	Thyroid imbalance disrupts progesterone levels.
	Miscarriage	Inadequate thyroid reserves to both nurture embryo and attend to body's needs; particularly common during winter months. Results in inadequate supply of progesterone to sustain pregnancy.
	Frequent colds and flus Difficulty in recovering from infection	Immune suppression due to low thyroid levels. Related autoimmune disorder, such as Hashimoto's.
	Abdominal cramping, diarrhea, constipation (IBS)	Reduced muscular activity of bowel walls due to thyroid depletion. Body fluid overload due to inadequate progesterone production premenstrually. PMS and diarrhea due to thyroid related hormonal dysregulation.
	PMS	Inadequate production of progesterone in the second half of the cycle.

Chapter 6

———— • ◆ • ————

Who's at Risk for Hypothyroidism?

Many permanent and temporary conditions can be at the root of hypothyroidism. The two most common causes are Hashimoto's thyroiditis, an autoimmune condition, and *over*treatment of *hyper*thyroidism (giving too much hormone-lowering drug). When problems come from the thyroid gland or thyroid hormone levels, the diagnosis is called primary hypothyroidism. In some cases, it is caused by disorders of the pituitary gland (in which case it is known as secondary hypothyroidism) or the hypothalamus gland (tertiary hypothyroidism).

The main causes of hypothyroidism are:

- Autoimmune thyroiditis, the most common type of hypothyroidism, is caused by an autoimmune dysfunction. Subtypes are Hashimoto's thyroiditis (the most prevalent), atrophic thyroiditis, and Riedel's thyroiditis.
- Mild hypothyroidism, also known as subclinical, sub-acute, evolving, and compensated hypothyroidism, is

marked by slightly elevated TSH levels but normal T4. Symptoms can be severe even with tests only slightly abnormal.

- Surgically induced hypothyroidism. Removal of the thyroid gland, usually due to cancer, will certainly result in hypothyroidism (see page 98).
- Treatment-induced hypothyroidism is caused by treatment of an overactive thyroid with medications or radioactive iodine (page 98).

Hypothyroidism also seems to arise with hallmark changes in life:

- Infancy. Congenital ("with birth") hypothyroidism occurs when a baby is born with low thyroid function or no thyroid gland due to genetic factors in the mother. (See chapter 9.)
- Teenage years. The hormonal advent of puberty, particularly in girls, can set in motion thyroid imbalances that manifest as fatigue, severe PMS, headaches, depression, and learning issues. (See chapter 10.)
- Pregnancy-induced hypothyroidism develops in women during pregnancy and manifests after delivery. (See chapter 8.)
- Age-induced hypothyroidism. As with most other body systems, the thyroid loses its potency as we age, making hypothyroidism a common trend in people over the age of sixty-five. (See chapter 13.)

It also appears that hypothyroidism results from other factors—or a combination of factors—which will be reported later in this chapter:

- Genetic factors. Researchers tell us that thyroid problems run in families. Scientists are hot on the trail of genetic links.
- Certain medications
- Environmental toxins (see chapter 14).

Even the foods we eat can play a role in hypothyroidism (see chapter 16). But one of the most common and difficult underlying risks is based in the body's defense system.

MEET YOUR IMMUNE SYSTEM

In previous chapters, the idea of an immune link with hypothyroidism has come up a number of times. We know that autoimmune thyroiditis (Hashimoto's) is the most common subtype. There also appears to be a link between immune dysfunction and other types of thyroiditis, including subclinical thyroiditis and pregnancy-induced thyroiditis—both of which may actually be manifestations of Hashimoto's. Autoimmune problems are implicated in failed or incomplete T4 to T3 conversion (see chapter 3), as well as associated syndromes such as fibromyalgia, hypoglycemia, and irritable bowel syndrome. In addition, it has been shown that people with one autoimmune disorder are at higher risk for others. We've talked about some of these theories in prior chapters, and will examine the others below. First, let's get better acquainted with the immune system and the process of autoimmunity.

A Mini-Lesson in Autoimmunity

The immune system is the body's defense team. It is a network of cells that guards the body against an outside world swarming with potential enemies—bacteria, viruses, fungi, and parasites. Under normal conditions, the immune system has a keen eye for detecting the difference between the cells that belong to the body and these potential threats. The cells in the body are marked with proteins that identify it as "self"; and as protein-carrying members of the body's union, these cells are protected from the immune system. Cells that lack the self-molecule are spotted by the immune system, which triggers an immune response. The "nonself" proteins are known as antigens. The word "antigen" derives from the Latin for "against a species."

When the immune system detects a virus or bacterium in the realm of the thyroid, it releases its (normally) well-trained defense system. The thyroid gland becomes inflamed, causing thyroiditis. Thyroiditis means inflammation ("itis") of the thyroid. "Inflammation" comes from the Latin verb meaning "to kindle or set on fire." An inflamed body part will swell and may produce liquids. Inflammation is one of the body's tactics for protecting itself from threatening outside forces. If you get a cold, your sinuses may become inflamed with immune products to fight off the bacteria. If you get a splinter, the area around it will swell and soften to encourage the expulsion of the unwanted inhabitant. An inflamed body part won't work as well as it normally does because it's busy fighting off the intruder.

However, inflammation can be triggered by more than just a dangerous outside invader. In fact, it is most often caused by a misguided immune system that turns its attack force against the very cells it is charged with protecting. When this happens on a regular basis, it is called an autoimmune disease. What does this mean?

In the case of thyroiditis, the body's own thyroid gland and/or hormones come under fire by antibodies. When antibodies attack the self, they are called autoantibodies. People with Hashimoto's thyroiditis, for example, have antibodies against cells in the thyroid. Antibodies in the blood can be detected by laboratory tests, and these tests are helpful in the diagnosis of autoimmune-based thyroid problems (see chapter 2). No one knows for sure why the immune system attacks the thyroid, but there are several theories.

Attack on the Transporting Proteins

As you might remember from chapter 3, more than 99 percent of T3 and T4 are bound to proteins called thyroglobulins, which usher them through the bloodstream. While they're tethered to thyroglobulin, thyroid hormones are inactive, locked in a protein stalemate. Only the freely circulating thyroid hormone (less than 1 percent) is biologically active. Over time, thyroid hormone is released at a controlled rate into the bloodstream.

This rate of thyroid hormone released from the proteins is dictated by the pituitary and TSH levels (see page 37), which send their messages to thyroid hormone by attaching to receptors. However, in people with Hashimoto's, the immune system's T cells attack the thyroid, triggering the release of excess protein. A posse of antibodies is then summoned to surround and cut off thyroglobulin supplies. Thyroglobulin is now perceived as being an outside invader—an antigen. The antigen blocks the TSH receptors on the thyroid, effectively limiting the amount of T4 that can be released and causing thyroid deficiency.

Genetics

There is also some evidence supporting a genetic predisposition to autoimmune disorders. Hashimoto's does have a tendency to cluster in families, but researchers are still searching for consistent genetic markers. About half of those with close relatives with chronic autoimmune disease have antibodies—the immune system's agents for attacking specific proteins—to the thyroid. As many as half of those with a common genetic disease of women called Turner's syndrome have hypothyroidism, usually resulting from Hashimoto's thyroiditis.

Stress

Research also supports the concept that ongoing stress can interfere with the normal functioning of the immune system and heighten an individual's vulnerability to autoimmune disease. It can disrupt the ability of the immune system to respond to anti-inflammatory signals. Some patients in my practice remember a highly stressful event—such as a car accident or the death of a loved one—preceding the onset of their hypothyroid symptoms.

Infection and Other Triggers

Some clinicians believe that autoimmune hypothyroidism is triggered by a previous infection, or even caused directly by an infection. For example, one study showed a link between hepatitis C and the onset of autoimmune disease.

There also seems to be a link between autoimmune thyroid disease and environmental toxins, such as insecticides, plastics, smoking, and soy products, called phytoestrogens—fake estrogens which, in the case of hypothyroidism, imitate estrogen, fatten up protein cells to bind with more T3/T4, and reduce the amount of active thyroid hormone in the body. Some believe that these xenoestrogens (another term for them, which means "outsider" estrogens) confuse the immune system so that it attacks the thyroid. (See chapter 14.)

Some classic medical studies suggest that some allergic disorders seemed to occur with increased frequency among patients with thyroid problems. Possibly due to the immune component, people with hypothyroidism appear to have a higher tendency for outbreaks of hives (red and itchy welts). Although they generally respond to treatment with antihistamines, more recent research implies that some people who test positive for thyroid antibodies (but normal TSH) could reduce the number of flare-ups with thyroid replacement.

The Autoimmune Epidemic

It was once thought that chronic (ongoing) autoimmune diseases were rare. But those who follow them closely claim that we are in an epidemic. Autoimmune diseases represent the fourth largest cause of disability among women in the United States.

Researchers are finding autoimmune causes for widespread conditions. And it appears that having one type of autoimmune disease invites a susceptibility to others. An estimated 25 percent of people with autoimmune thyroid disease may develop other autoimmune conditions. Some common examples of these autoimmune diseases are rheumatoid arthritis (the immune cells attack the joints) and diabetes (the immune cells attack the pancreas, which produces insulin). About 10 percent of people with type I or juvenile diabetes mellitus develop chronic thyroiditis during their lives.

Women Are at Highest Risk

Hypothyroidism does not observe discrimination laws. Women are nine times more likely to get hypothyroidism. Three-fourths of autoimmune diseases in general strike women. And both tend to strike during the childbearing years (ages fourteen to forty-five). This has led experts to believe that female hormones (e.g., estrogen and progesterone) play a role in hypothyroidism. Men, children, and the elderly are not magically protected, but it occurs less often.

The most common autoimmune diseases of the thyroid are Hashimoto's thyroiditis, atrophic thyroiditis, and postpartum thyroiditis.

Diseases of the Thyroid

Hashimoto's Thyroiditis

Hashimoto's, the most common form of hypothyroidism in the United States, is a genetic disease named after the Japanese physician who first described it. Women are up to fifty times more likely to develop Hashimoto's thyroiditis than men and seven to ten times more likely to develop a related type of thyroid dysfunction called Graves' disease. The inflammation causes the thyroid gland to grow, forming a goiter, a fibrous growth in the neck that looks like a roll of fat. Like other forms of hypothyroidism, Hashimoto's thyroiditis requires lifelong treatment.

In early phases of the disease, there may be no symptoms at all, or a temporary period of *hyper*thyroidism (including feeling warm, diarrhea, anxiety, rapid heartbeat, unexplained weight loss). The attack on the thyroid causes an initial inflammatory response, which stimulates the thyroid to produce more hormone, which is why some people first become hyperthyroid with Hashimoto's. After a while, the thyroid starts to fail and becomes unable to respond to the signals from the pituitary to pump up production (see chapter 2). Hallmark symptoms are:

- Goiter (enlarged thyroid gland which may cause a bulge in the neck)
- Other endocrine disorders, such as diabetes, an underactive adrenal gland, and other autoimmune disorders
- Symptoms of hypothyroidism (see table on page 85) with an emphasis on fatigue, muscle weakness, and weight gain

My treatment of autoimmune thyroiditis, like other hypothyroid conditions, is based on physiologic 98 percent T4 and 2 percent T3.

Atrophic Thyroiditis

Atrophic thyroiditis is similar to Hashimoto's thyroiditis, except for the absence of a goiter.

Riedel's Thyroiditis

In a rare autoimmune disorder known as Riedel's thyroiditis, patients develop a hard stony mass that suggests cancer, but the disorder responds well to thyroid replacement and steroids.

De Quervain's Thyroiditis

De Quervain's thyroiditis (also called granulomatous thyroiditis) is much less common than Hashimoto's thyroiditis. The thyroid gland generally swells rapidly and is very painful and tender. The gland discharges thyroid hormone into the blood, and the patient becomes hyperthyroid; however, the gland quits taking up iodine (radioactive iodine uptake is very low), and the hyperthyroidism generally resolves over the next several weeks. In this condition, TSH levels are often high. A few patients will become hypothyroid once the inflammation settles down and will therefore need to stay on thyroid hormone replacement indefinitely.

Silent Thyroiditis

Silent thyroiditis was not recognized until the 1970s, although it probably existed and was treated as Graves' disease before that. This type of thyroiditis is a hybrid of Hashimoto's thyroiditis and de Quervain's thyroiditis. Its laboratory profile is similar to de Quervain's (high TSH, low radioactive iodine uptake), but biopsy of the gland with needle aspiration reveals cells that look like those in Hashimoto's disease. Young postpartum women are most susceptible. No treatment is usually needed, since 80 percent of patients recover within three months. The thyroid gland is only slightly larger. Rarely, patients become irreversibly hypothyroid and need to be placed on thyroid hormone.

Mild Hypothyroidism

Mild hypothyroidism (also known as "subclinical," "compensated," or "evolving" hypothyroidism) is a condition in which T4 levels are normal but TSH levels are elevated, and the patient experiences symptoms ranging from mild to severe. Untreated patients carry an increased risk of heart disease, high lipids, miscarriage, and a host of other hypothyroid-related problems that are "silent" but potentially deadly.

In a landmark study of subclinical hypothyroidism in which 2,779 patients were followed for twenty years, the investigators concluded that women with both increased TSH levels and thyroid antibodies had the highest risk of hypothyroidism. For women with subclinical hypothyroidism but without thyroid antibodies, the risk was about four times lower; and so was the risk of hypothyroidism in women with thyroid antibodies and *normal* TSH concentrations. As we saw in chapter 2, this large-scale study, reported in the *British Medical Journal* in 1997, called into question the widely accepted laboratory reference range for "normal": ". . . even within the reference range of around 0.5–4.5 mU/l, a high thyroid stimulating hormone concentration (>2 mU/l) was associated with an increased risk of future hypothyroidism."

Pregnancy-Induced Thyroiditis

Pregnancy-induced thyroiditis tends to arise in the first few months after a woman has delivered a baby (the postpartum period), but it can start during pregnancy, when it may pose risks to the fetus. The nurturing of a growing fetus requires an enormous reserve of thyroid from the pregnant mother. I believe that many women, particularly in geographic areas subject to distinct seasonal changes, do not have the necessary thyroid reserve to carry a fetus to term without suffering some level of thyroid depletion. Thyroid imbalances can sometimes cause unexplained infertility or miscarriages, particularly early in pregnancy. Women should therefore be monitored closely. (See chapter 8.)

Age-Induced Hypothyroidism

Age-induced hypothyroidism is particularly common in women over the age of fifty, when many body systems begin to slow down naturally. An estimated 10 percent of women over the age of fifty show signs of a failing thyroid. After the age of sixty-five, the ratio of women to men evens out. (See chapter 13.)

Surgery-Induced Hypothyroidism

A thyroid disorder such as thyroid cancer may warrant partial or complete removal of the thyroid, causing hypothyroidism and necessitating hormone replacement. Regular follow-up to gauge thyroid function is critical.

Treatment-Induced Hypothyroisism

Some forms of hyperthyroidism, such as Graves' disease, are treated with radioactive iodine. This treatment destroys over-active thyroid cells but usually results in hypothyroidism. However, hypothyroidism may not occur for months or years after radioactive iodine treatment ends, making the link between symptoms (usually weight gain, fatigue, brain fog) and hypothyroidism difficult. For this reason, regular thyroid check-ups should be scheduled to monitor your thyroid health.

Thyroid Nodules and Cancer

A thyroid nodule is a lump or growth in your thyroid gland. Functioning nodules act like thyroid glands and produce thyroid hormones. Many thyroid nodules never cause problems and go undetected by both patients and doctors. However, about 10 percent of thyroid nodules are cancerous. The good news is that the survival rate is high with early detection and treatment.

When a thyroid nodule is found (usually during a routine office visit), you will probably undergo several tests to determine if the nodule is cancerous and whether it requires treatment. These tests may include:

- A TSH test to determine the amount of thyroid-stimulating hormone in your bloodstream

- An ultrasound to show the exact size and location of the nodule
- A biopsy to determine if the thyroid nodule is benign or cancerous

Your doctor may prescribe thyroid hormone tablets to try to shrink a noncancerous nodule. You will need to be tested periodically to see if your thyroid has shrunk, to be sure that your thyroid-stimulating hormone is in the proper range, and to adjust the dosage of your thyroid hormone. If the nodule does not respond to treatment or continues to grow, your doctor may recommend that it be removed surgically.

Even suspicious nodules can turn out to be benign. But if a nodule is cancerous, your doctor will recommend immediate removal of the thyroid, or part of it. Hypothyroidism will most likely result, and with it the need for thyroid hormone replacement.

Autoimmune Clusters

There are more than eighty autoimmune diseases. If you have one type of autoimmune disease, you or someone in your family is at higher risk of having another. Though most autoimmune conditions are relatively rare, several, including rheumatoid arthritis, autoimmune thyroid disease, systemic lupus erythematosus, and diabetes, are fairly prevalent. Hormonal, genetic, and environmental factors may be at play in causing diseases of different types to cluster in families. In addition to the disorders described below, the misdirected immune system can attack virtually any part of the body, including the blood vessels and the skin, causing a number of symptoms. Fibromyalgia and irritable bowel syndrome are thought to have an autoimmune component; they're described in more depth in chapter 5. I refer you to

Mary J. Shomon's book *Living Well with Autoimmune Disease* and her Web site at www.thyroid-info.com on this issue (see Resources at the back of this book).

Autoimmune Disorder	Symptoms	Treatment
Autoimmune thyroiditis—immune system destroys the thyroid	Mental and physical sluggishness, sensitivity to cold, weight gain, coarsening of the skin, goiter	Thyroid hormone replacement
Guillain-Barré syndrome—immune attack of nerves primarily instigated by viral infection	Tingling in the fingers and toes, muscle weakness, difficulty in breathing, and, in advanced cases, paralysis	Supportive care (whirlpools, plasmapheresis—removal of antibody-laden plasma)
Inflammatory bowel syndrome (IBS)—autoimmune attack of the lining of the lower GI tract	Diarrhea (sometimes bloody), ulcers on skin, abdominal cramps, joint pains, and fatigue	Symptom relief with antidiarrhea medication; corticosteroids to reduce inflammation; surgery in advanced cases to remove affected section of bowel
Insulin-dependent (type I) diabetes—inflammation of pancreas resulting in reduced insulin production and excess glucose	Increased thirst and urination, nausea and vomiting, fatigue, weight loss, proneness to infections.	Insulin therapy and diet modification
Multiple sclerosis—inflammation of nerves	Tingling/numbness in arms and legs, trembling, impaired vision, difficulty in walking, spasticity	Corticosteroids for inflammation, interferon, bacofen
Myasthenia gravis—autoimmune attack of the muscles	Muscle weakness; difficulty in breathing, talking, swallowing; double vision and drooping eyelids	Edrophonium and daily rest
Rheumatoid arthritis—inflammation of the membrane around joints, and the heart, lungs, and/or eyes	Inflamed and/or deformed joints, loss of strength, swelling, pain	Bed rest, exercise of affected joint, anti-inflammatory drugs for relief of pain and swelling

Autoimmune Disorder	Symptoms	Treatment
Scleroderma—activation of immune cells which results in scar tissue in the skin, internal organs, and small blood vessels	*Raynaud's phenomenon (extreme sensitivity to cold in hands and feet), swelling of the fingers/hands, skin thickening, skin ulcers, joint stiffness in the hands, sore throat, diarrhea*	*Symptomatic treatment of each affected body system*
Sjögren's syndrome/disease—inability to secrete tears and saliva	*Dry gritty eyes and dry mouth, dental caries, swollen glands*	*Artificial tears, hydration by drinking lots of water*
Systemic lupus erythematosus—inflammation of the connective tissues	*Fever, weight loss, hair loss, mouth and nose sores, malaise, fatigue, seizures, symptoms of mental illness; 50 percent develop a classic "butterfly" rash across the nose and cheeks; 20 percent have Raynaud's phenomenon (extreme sensitivity to cold in hands and feet)*	*Anti-inflammatory drugs, such as oral corticosteroids, and antimalarial drugs*

IMPACT OF DRUGS

As a side effect, some drugs have a negative impact on thyroid function. These include amiodarone (used for serious cardiac arrhythmias), lithium (for bipolar disorder), iodine (table salt), and antithyroid drugs.

LOW IODINE

Insufficient iodine leads to a decrease in thyroid hormones. The manifestations of low iodine levels are grouped together under the name iodine deficiency disorder (IDD). These disorders include goiter (enlarged thyroid gland), hypothyroidism, mental retardation, reproductive problems, and a wide range of neurological and physical disorders.

The body does not produce iodine; it must be consumed in the diet. IDD arises when there is not enough iodine in the soil, which impacts the water we drink (groundwater leaches iodine), the crops we eat (food grown in iodine-poor soil), and meats we consume (from animals grazing on the land).

As we learned in chapter 2, the thyroid gland extracts iodine from the bloodstream and uses it to make T4 and T3. Goiter may be the first symptom of mild iodine deficiency. Hypothyroidism may also result. Goiters can lead to functioning thyroid nodules and hyperthyroidism. The most critical damage is to developing embryos, infants, and young children nurtured by mothers who consume insufficient iodine. Undetected hypothyroidism in the first months of life can cause irreversible brain damage and lower intelligence later in life. The impact of early hypothyroidism will be discussed in chapter 9.

A very small amount of iodine packs a wallop. A teaspoon supplies your *lifetime* needs. But the body can't store iodine, so it must be replenished regularly. A pinch of iodized salt a day should keep deficiency away.

Chapter 7

I Suspect I Have
Hypothyroidism Because . . .

As you read this book, you may recognize yourself in the case studies. You may find that what you learn jogs your memory about family history, symptoms, environmental exposures, or prescription drugs that could impact your test results or your treatment. Use this work sheet to collect your thoughts—and to focus them for your next office visit.

Name: _____

Age:_____

Gender: _____

Married: yes ☐ no ☐

Children:

_____

_____

Illnesses and dates diagnosed:

_____

_____

_____

_____

_____

_____

Prior surgery:

_____

_____

_____

I have the following hypothyroid symptoms	When symptoms are most likely to occur (time of day, month, year)
Skin and outer body:	
Dry skin	
Coarse skin	
Coarse, brittle hair	
Hair loss	
Nail weakness/thinness	
Edema (swelling) of eyelids	
Sensation of cold	
Cold skin	
Decreased sweating	
Pallid skin	
Generalized:	
Weakness	
Insomnia	
Lethargy	
Slow speech	
Thick tongue	
Headaches/migraines	
Muscles and joints:	
Muscle weakness	
Muscle pain	

I have the following hypothyroid symptoms	When symptoms are most likely to occur (time of day, month, year)
Carpal tunnel	
Fibromyalgia	
Swelling of hands/feet	
Gastrointestinal:	
Irritable bowel syndrome	
Abdominal pain	
Cramping	
Diarrhea (especially near time of menstrual flow)	
Constipation	
Unexplained gain in weight	
Loss/gain in appetite	
Hormonal/reproductive:	
PMS	
Excessive menstruation	
Lack of menstruation (amenorrhea)	
Menopausal symptoms (hot flashes, etc.)	
Infertility	
Frequent miscarriage	
Loss of libido	
Emotional/mental:	
Brain fog	
Memory loss	
Panic attacks	
Depression	
Change in personality—less outgoing, less joyful	
Seasonal affective disorder (depression during winter months)	
Cardiac:	
High blood pressure	
Palpitations	
Heart click (mitral valve prolapse)	
Pain in the chest wall	
Heart enlargement (congestive heart failure)	

I have the following hypothyroid symptoms	When symptoms are most likely to occur (time of day, month, year)
High lipids	
Cholesterol	
LDL/triglycerides	
Homocysteine	
Low HDL	

Recent stresses/concerns:

_____

_____

_____

_____

_____

_____

Close relatives who have been diagnosed with thyroid disease: hypothyroidism, hyperthyroidism, Graves' disease, thyroid nodules, goiter, thyroid cancer:

☐ Mother: _____

☐ Father: _____

☐ Siblings: _____

☐ Other (aunts, uncles, cousins, grandparents):_____

IS AUTOIMMUNE DISEASE IN YOUR FAMILY?

Until recently, awareness of autoimmune disease was low. If family photos of Great-Aunt Sally show her with a funny rash over her face and she was known to get tired a lot, doctors didn't know whether it was lupus. That's why I've provided clues—telltale signs to help you unravel some of the medical mysteries in your family that might support your hypothyroidism diagnosis.

Type of Autoimmune Disease	Who Might Have It (including you)	Definite Diagnosis or Suspicion
Anemia *Clue:* skin pallor and extreme weakness		☐ Diagnosed ☐ Suspected
Diabetes (type I, insulin dependent) *Clue:* frequent urination, weight loss, increased thirst		☐ Diagnosed ☐ Suspected
Endometriosis *Clue:* severe menstrual cramps and/or infertility		☐ Diagnosed ☐ Suspected
Multiple sclerosis *Clue:* muscle spasticity		☐ Diagnosed ☐ Suspected
Myasthenia gravis *Clue:* muscle weakness		☐ Diagnosed ☐ Suspected
Raynaud's syndrome *Clue:* extreme cold intolerance		☐ Diagnosed ☐ Suspected
Rheumatoid arthritis *Clue:* stiff joints		☐ Diagnosed ☐ Suspected
Sjögren's syndrome *Clue:* dry eyes and mouth		☐ Diagnosed ☐ Suspected
Systemic lupus erythematosus *Clue:* "butterfly" rash over the nose and cheeks		☐ Diagnosed ☐ Suspected
Vitiligo *Clue:* white or red patches on skin		☐ Diagnosed ☐ Suspected

I've been exposed to the following goitrogens:

☐ soy consumption _____ times a day

Please describe your soy diet:

_____

_____

☐ drug therapy with lithium, amiodarone, thyroid-reducing drugs

Other drug therapy:

_____

_____

☐ cigarettes (smoker/secondary smoke)

What stands out about your family's medical history? List anything you think might be relevant.

Maternal grandparent: _____

Medical history: _____

_____

_____

Maternal grandparent: _____

Medical history: _____

_____

_____

Paternal grandparent: _____

Medical history: _____

_____

_____

Paternal grandparent: _____

Medical history: _____

_____

_____

Parent: _____

Medical history: _____

_____

_____

Parent: _____

Medical history: _____

_____

_____

My name: _____

Medical history: _____

_____

_____

Sibling: _____

Medical history: _____

_____

_____

Sibling: _____

Medical history: _____

_____

_____

Sibling: _____

Medical history: _____

_____

_____

Child: _____

Medical history: _____

_____

_____

Child: _____

Medical history: _____

_____

_____

Child:_____

Medical history: _____

_____

_____

Child: _____

Medical history: _____

_____

_____

BIBLIOGRAPHY ABSTRACTS

Your doctor may want to know about my approach to hypothyroidism. What follows are brief reviews of some of the more important studies mentioned in the preceding chapters.

Thyroid levels above 2.0 μU/ml (mU/l)
indicate hypothyroidism risk.

The spectrum of thyroid disease in a community: The Whickham survey. 1977. *Clin Endocrinol* 7:481–93.

This study and the twenty-year follow-up study published in the *British Medical Journal* yielded invaluable data on the natural history of thyroid disorders. A main conclusion of the study was that thyroid-stimulating hormone concentrations above 2.0 mU/l are associated with an increased risk of hypothyroidism. Half of the study population (male and female) fall into this category. This conclusion was based on the change in the slope of the line obtained when the log of the serum thyroid-stimulating hormone concentration was related to the probability of developing hypothyroidism over a twenty-year period in women. The probability of a forty-year-old woman with a thyroid-stimulating hormone of 2.1 mU/l developing hypothyroidism is low: one in fifty over twenty years. In men, the probability is so low that an equivalent could not be derived.

Patients are not well controlled on T4.

Colorado Thyroid Disease Prevalence Study Archives of Internal Medicine 2000. 160:526–34.

Thyroid dysfunction may be more common than previously appreciated. In a study of 25,862 patients attending a state health fair, the prevalence of elevated TSH determinations was about 9.5 percent, and approximately 2 percent of patients had a low TSH. Surprisingly, among patients on *l*-thyroxine with known thyroid disease, 40 percent had abnormal TSH determinations.

Subclinical hypothyroidism is common and should be treated.
Weetman, A. P. Fortnightly review: Hypothyroidism: screen-ing and subclinical disease. 1997. *BMJ* 314 (Apr. 19): 1175.
This meta-analysis yielded the following conclusions:

- Subclinical hypothyroidism is common, especially in elderly women.
- The presence of subclinical hypothyroidism or thyroid antibodies increases the risk of developing overt hypothy-roidism, and the risk is even greater (about 5 percent a year) if both are present together.
- Thyroid-stimulating hormone concentrations above 2.0 mU/l are associated with an increased risk of hypothy-roidism.
- Screening all acutely ill patients or the healthy general population for hypothyroidism is not recommended. Case finding, especially in women over forty with non-specific symptoms, is currently the best approach to de-tect previously unsuspected hypothyroidism.
- Modest symptomatic benefits occur with thyroxine treat-ment in some patients with subclinical hypothyroidism, and lipid profiles may also improve.
- Monitored thyroxine treatment, maintaining normal thyroid-stimulating hormone concentrations, has no ad-verse effects.

T3 conversion may vary at the tissue level (liver).
J Clin Endocrinol Metab 1993. 77:1431–35. ". . . [this study] shows that transport of thyroid hormone may vary at the tissue level. Furthermore, as T3 is the principal biologically active thyroid hormone, regulation of transport of T3 into the REP may play a (patho)physiological role in the ultimate de-termination of thyroid hormone activity in the tissues."

Smoking raises the risk of hypothyroidism.

Smoking as a risk factor for Graves' disease, toxic nodular goiter, and autoimmune hypothyroidism. 2002. *Thyroid* 12 (1) (Jan.): 69–75.

T3 helps hasten response to antidepressants.

Does thyroid supplementation accelerate tricyclic antidepressant response? A review and meta-analysis of the literature. 2001. *Am J Psychiatry* 158 (10) (Oct.): 1617–22.

There is some evidence, from a small number of randomized trials, that patients with depression who receive treatment with tricyclic antidepressants will have a more favorable response if they are also treated with T3. The benefit, in some patients, appears to come in the form of a more rapid response to the antidepressant medication, which can normally take four to eight weeks to exert a beneficial therapeutic response. Not all the T3-treated patients show benefit, and the risks of T3 supplementation must be carefully assessed, versus the potential benefit in each patient.

Hypothyroidism in pregnancy causes lower IQ in children.

National Institutes of Child Health and Human Development (NICHD) and Dr. James Haddow reported the following in the August 19, 2002, issue of the *New England Journal of Medicine:*

Children born to mothers with untreated hypothyroidism during pregnancy score lower on IQ tests than children of healthy mothers. However, children whose mothers were being treated for the condition scored almost the same as children born to healthy mothers. These findings suggest that early detection and treatment of hypothyroidism in pregnant women are a critical part of prenatal care.

Hypothyroidism during pregnancy raises risk of neonatal heart defects.

Wolfberg, A. J., and D. A. Nagey. Thyroid disease during pregnancy and subsequent congenital anomalies. 2002. Abstract #274. Annual meeting of the Society for Maternal-Fetal Medicine in New Orleans, Jan. 17.

The researchers studied 101 women (some with hypothyroidism and others with hyperthyroidism) who gave birth at the Johns Hopkins Hospital between December 1994 and June 1999. The women's average age was thirty-one; very few admitted to smoking, drinking alcohol, or using illegal drugs. Overall, there were 108 pregnancies with 114 fetuses. The research team studied the charts for all children born from these pregnancies and recorded any medical problems during the neonatal period or subsequent years.

Twenty-one babies (18 percent) had birth defects, including problems in the cardiac, renal, and central nervous systems and other disorders such as sunken chest, extra fingers, cleft lip and palate, and ear deformities. Two fetuses died before being delivered. Among a subset of 86 women who had a test of their thyroid function performed during the first trimester of pregnancy (52 with hypothyroidism and 34 with hyperthyroidism), 17 babies (20 percent) had medical problems similar to those seen among the larger group. The women with hypothyroidism were more likely than those with hyperthyroidism to have babies with defects. The authors say it is possible that the same antibodies that cause the underactive thyroid could also be responsible for the birth defects.

10–15 percent of clinically depressed suffer from hypothyroidism.

Twenty million Americans have thyroid disease. 1996. Rev. 1 (3) (May): *American Thyroid Association*

- Most patients with hypothyroidism have some degree of depression, ranging from mild to severe.
- Ten to 15 percent of the patients with a diagnosis of depression may have thyroid hormone deficiency.
- Patients with depression should be tested to determine if they have a thyroid disorder.

T3 helps improve cognitive function.

Impairment in cognitive and exercise performance during prolonged Antarctic residence: Effect of supplementation in the polar triiodothyronine syndrome. 2001. *J Clin Endocrinol Metab* 86:110–16.

The Antarctic study, conducted by Dr. H. Lester Reed and colleagues, measured the thyroid hormone levels in twelve adult individuals while they were living in Antarctica. The study began when the subjects arrived there, and it lasted for eleven months. During the first four months (period 1), while all the subjects received a daily placebo, the pooled value for thyroid hormone levels in all the subjects dropped significantly, as did their moods and their performance on tests of mental skills and exercise capacity. At the beginning of the fifth month, half the subjects began receiving daily T3 supplements instead of the placebo, while the other half continued to receive a placebo.

At the end of that month, and for the following six months (period 2), during which the supplementation continued, the test group showed a marked improvement in cognitive performance above the baseline measurements. The control group, however, remained below baseline in their measurements of cognitive performance after the fifth month. Depressive symptoms remained higher in both groups during period 2, compared with baseline, but the test group reported significantly less fatigue/inertia and confusion/bewilderment than the control group during this period.

T3 elevates mood.

Bunevicius, R., and A. J. Prange. *Int J Neuropsychopharmacol* 3 2000. (2) (June): 167–74.

The authors treated twenty-six hypothyroid women—eleven with autoimmune thyroiditis and fifteen who had been treated for thyroid cancer—with their usual dose of T4 or with a regimen in which 50 mcg of T4 had been replaced by 12.5 mcg of T3. Patients were first randomly assigned to one regimen for five weeks and then to a second regimen for an additional five weeks. The substitution of T3 for a portion of T4 caused expected changes in concentrations of thyroid hormones and TSH. After combined hormone treatment, there were clear improvements in both cognition and mood, the latter changes being greater. The patients who had been treated for thyroid cancer showed more mental improvement than the women with autoimmune thyroiditis, perhaps because they were more dependent on exogenous hormone. Some mood improvements correlated positively with changes in TSH, while others correlated negatively with changes in free T4.

T2 may be an active metabolite.

Demonstration of *in vitro* metabolic effects of 3,5 diiodothyronine. *Gen Comp Endocrinol* 104 1996. (1) (Oct.): 61–66.

". . . results suggest that 3,5-T(2) exerts metabolic effects on energy expenditure, on both lipid beta-oxidation and leucine metabolism in hypothyroid rats. We conclude that 3,5 T(2) is a metabolically active iodothyronine."

PART II

Mastering Your
Thyroid Rhythms
at Every Stage of Life

As the body's instrument of change, thyroid hormone helps your body and mind to keep pace with the varied metabolic challenges that come your way from infancy to old age. In the previous section, we looked at the nitty-gritty science behind my approach with the Two-Week Diagnostic Trial and the combination of 2 percent T3 with 98 percent T4. In part II, we'll see how these strategies apply successfully at different stages of life—each of which presents its own unique challenges.

We'll start with pregnancy, the time when symptoms often first arise. If you are a mother, father, or close relative with hypothyroidism, it behooves you to keep a close watch on the children in your life for subtle signs. The enormous demands on thyroid hormone during this time of rapid growth can quickly drain thyroid reserves. You'll see the real value of a Two-Week Diagnostic Trial (modulated to the special needs of individuals) as a safe way of confirming or ruling out hypothyroidism—or ruling out other conditions such as attention deficit disorder, one of hypothyroidism—or ruling out other conditions such as attention deficit disorder, one of hypothyroidism's look-alikes in young children.

Some people can hum along for years with no problem, then, suddenly, with perimenopausal symptoms comes hypothyroidism. Alternately, most hypothroid patients respond well to the same T4 or T4/T3 combination dosage for long periods, but then many of them require adjustments as the metabolic rhythms of their lives demand significant changes in thyroid hormone. Puberty and menopause frame the reproductive years—they're times of physical or emotional stress that can throw hormones off balance. From inception to advanced age, I will explain the subtle and obvious milestones that disrupt hormonal rhythms, and how to recognize these changes, and give you the vocabulary for discussing the need for adjustments with your doctor.

Chapter 8

In the Beginning
There Was Hypothyroidism:
Fertility, Pregnancy, and Beyond

When Ruth, aged thirty-two, first came to see me, she said that she felt great, and she looked fine—only slight eyebrow thinning. There was just one thing wrong, and it was consuming her: She couldn't get pregnant. In fact, it was an infertility workup that first unmasked her thyroid problem.

When first diagnosed, Ruth described herself as always having "the highest energy level of anyone I know," so she was perplexed by her borderline-high TSH (6.3). But she also reported that both her mother and grandmother took thyroid hormone for hypothyroidism. Her previous doctor had given her 25 mcg of Levoxyl (T4). The T4 regimen had lowered her TSH to within normal limits (1.99), and her free T4 levels were normal.

As an aside, it should be noted that high TSH without significant symptoms is not uncommon. The condition is called subclinical hypothyroidism, or mild hypothyroidism (chapter

6), which can represent an early, or "evolving," form of thyroid disease, particularly autoimmune hypothyroidism (Hashimoto's). There's much debate in the medical community about whether subclinical hypothyroidism should be treated. The main reason for doing so is to prevent "silent" serious symptoms such as cardiovascular disease in older women. In this case, Ruth's silent problem was infertility.

A little deeper into our discussion I gained more insight into the source of Ruth's infertility. While she never had significant problems with PMS, she always had very scant periods that lasted nine or ten days, and sometimes she skipped months. After going off birth control, she did not have a spontaneous period for eight months (amenorrhea), at which point she was artificially cycled with progestin.

My first goal was to achieve a physiologic balance of T4/T3 levels by changing her Levoxyl dose to one-half a 50-mcg tablet a day (for a total daily dose of 25 mcg), except on Mondays and Fridays, when she received a full dose, and added time-release T3 to her existing regimen.

The Levoxyl change raised Ruth's T4 dose somewhat and eliminated the yellow dye that is present in the 25-mcg tablet. In addition, the introduction of a physiologic level of T3 in time-release form actually increases the need for T4, which is a major factor accounting for the spotty results seen by many physicians who have tried T3 in the past few years.

After several months without success on this regimen, I replaced synthetic T3 with natural thyroid extract in a time-release capsule and readjusted the Levoxyl dose to physiologic proportions: 98 percent T4 and 2 percent T3. By June, much to our collective joy, Ruth was pregnant.

I've monitored Ruth's TSH levels closely (they tend to rise during pregnancy). Her dosages were increased slightly on several occasions during pregnancy to maintain an adequate reserve. And at this writing, she is seven months pregnant and doing well: no fatigue, no acid reflux. And she continues to work full-time at her job.

Success stories like Ruth's illustrate some important learnings I'd like to pass along about hypothyroidism and pregnancy.

CORRECT MENSTRUAL PROBLEMS TODAY FOR FERTILITY TOMORROW

In hypothyroidism, normal hormonal rhythms of estrogen and progesterone and other hormones go awry. Fluctuating estrogen levels wreak havoc with thyroid hormone. As you might remember from chapter 2, estrogen tends to increase the levels of proteins that ferry thyroid hormone through the blood and store it for future use. While hitching onto the protein, the thyroid hormone is inactive. If there's too much protein, then there's less "free" thyroid hormone available to do its metabolic job. As a result, many of my younger female patients come to me with severe PMS or irregular periods or very heavy periods—all signs of a hormonal system in chaos.

Reported estimates of menstrual irregularities in hypothyroid women range from 23 to 70 percent. I think these estimates are vastly underestimated because they're based on patients having abnormal TSH levels, which of course many hypothyroid women do not.

The most common problem is oligomenorrhea, scant or infrequent menstruation. Severe hypothyroidism is linked with failure to ovulate, or anovulation. In mild hypothyroidism, ovulation and conception can occur, but when thyroid reserves are low, there's a higher chance of miscarriage, stillbirth, or prematurity. Six out of every one hundred miscarriages can be attributed to thyroid deficiency during pregnancy. But there again the relationship is underestimated, since the thyroid status of the women having miscarriages will be defined by their TSH results.

Take Action

Recognize menstrual problems, especially failure to ovulate, as a possible indicator of hypothyroidism and future fertility problems. You may be able to set a clock by your periods and still not be ovulating. To find out, test your ovulation with over-the-counter tests for a few months in a row. Follow up with a thyroid exam and treatment to correct the problem.

CHECK YOUR AUTOIMMUNE STATUS

Having preexisting autoimmune thyroiditis (Hashimoto's) is a double-edged sword during pregnancy. On the one hand, pregnancy can send your symptoms into a heavenly state of remission; the immune system during pregnancy is much depressed in order to accept the developing fetus. On the other hand, Hashimoto's raises your risk of a miscarriage because it may be reducing the thyroid reserve needed to compensate (thyroidwise) as the pregnancy progresses.

Some but not all studies show that women with confirmed Hashimoto's have higher incidences of infertility, miscarriage, and premature delivery. More women with endometriosis (29 percent) had positive antibodies than others. In one study, 18 percent of women with a positive thyroid peroxidase antibody (TPO-Ab)—the diagnostic test for Hashimoto's—were infertile, compared to just 8 percent of women without thyroid disease. The studies that link Hashimoto's to these problems make the fundamental assumption (wrong in my opinion) that since TSH results are the same in both groups, thyroid function is also the same—and pregnancy problems must be fundamentally due to immunologic problems. It's important not to jump to conclusions based on the flawed assumption that the thyroid metabolic status of a group of individuals is absolutely defined by the average TSH of that group.

Remember also that the presence of thyroid antibodies increases the risk of developing overt hypothyroidism in people with mild (subclinical) hypothyroidism, about 5 percent a year.

Women with antithyroid antibodies not only have trouble conceiving, they may be more prone to miscarriage. They often have antibodies to phospholipids, which are important components in the blood vessel walls of the placenta. These antibodies can cut off blood flow in the placenta, resulting in pregnancy loss.

Take Action

Infertile women with suspected hypothyroidism should have both their TSH and their TPO-Ab levels checked. A TSH alone might not be able to detect what the TPO-Ab can: an early and evolving case of autoimmune thyroiditis. And, as we'll see in the next section, sufficient treatment is critical to both conception and the developing baby.

If an immune cause for pregnancy loss is identified, you and your doctor should discuss the benefits of treatment with heparin and aspirin, white-cell immunization, high-dose progesterone, or intravenous immune globulin. Immunotherapy is controversial, and while many studies offer promise, the experimental data have not shown conclusively whether any of these immunotherapies are effective.

IF YOU BECOME PREGNANT . . .

The effects of pregnancy on thyroid reserve are so great that nearly one out of fifty women in the United States is diagnosed with hypothyroidism during pregnancy. Here are some ways to help ensure that you are properly diagnosed—and treated. Treatment is important not only to prevent miscarriage (which is more likely in women with hypothyroidism) but also to help safeguard the mental and physical health of your child at birth and throughout life.

Thyroid Hormone Is Natural and Necessary

Many women are concerned about taking anything "unnatural" during pregnancy out of fear of hurting their babies. Fear not. Thyroid hormone *is* a natural entity—not a foreign drug with the potential for unknown toxicity. I do recommend dosage forms of synthetic hormone that are as free of excipients and dyes as possible to avoid allergic reactions in the mother. The key is to arrive at the most physiologic dose, which in my practice is the 2 percent solution—2 percent T3 and 98 percent T4. This proportion reflects healthy hormone levels, which are what's needed to optimize healthy baby development.

Make sure that other factors don't interfere with or enhance thyroid absorption. Many prenatal vitamin pills, for example, contain iron, which interferes with thyroid absorption. The amount of iron in a prenatal vitamin is small compared to iron capsules your doctor may prescribe if you're iron-deficient. The iron capsules should always be separated from thyroid by taking them with the evening meal. I suggest taking the prenatal vitamins at lunch, with thyroid taken first thing in the morning before breakfast. Fiber can also reduce thyroid absorption, so if more fiber is specifically needed for constipation, you need to allow more time for the thyroid hormone to be absorbed before breakfast.

All things considered, I do not believe we should overworry such issues, since the thyroid doses will need to be adjusted anyway in the course of the pregnancy, and adjusting your dosage on the basis of how you feel will compensate for changes in thyroid hormone absorption.

Make Sure Your TSH Is in the Mid to Low Range

Your TSH may be normal according to your local lab, but it may not be "normal enough" to maintain a pregnancy. Because of the higher metabolic demands of pregnancy, more thyroid hormone needs to be available. Many reference labs consider a range of 0.4 to 5.0 as normal, although some labs have narrowed the range to 0.4 to 3.0. But is a level of 3.0 low enough to carry a pregnancy? I do not believe so. I would err on a lower TSH (below 2.0), due to the higher demand, to encourage pregnancy.

CONSIDER SEASONAL ISSUES

Only a handful of women have enough thyroid reserve to remain fully compensated thyroidwise throughout a pregnancy in a cold climate. The twin burdens of pregnancy and hypothyroidism bring out symptoms, and the additional burden of cold weather further drains thyroid reserves.

Hypothyroidism is so seasonally related that women are at their peak status right at the end of summer, so they're more likely to get pregnant then. When they get to November, they're three months pregnant. At this point, the thyroid demand is higher because of seasonal change: Cold weather re-

---

Take Action

If your doctor refuses to treat you because your TSH levels are normal, and you still have not conceived, point out the study mentioned on pages 122–123 and the instability of the "normal" range by clinical authorities—or find a doctor with a more liberal treatment philosophy (see chapter 18). Remember these points:

- The AACE recently revised its definition of normal, now recommending treatment above 3.0 (not 5.5 as before).
- The *British Medical Journal* assures, and I wholeheartedly agree, that there's no harm in treating at TSH levels of 2.0.
- Thyroid demands are higher in patients wishing to conceive and carry a pregnancy, so TSH levels should be lower.

---

quires more thyroid hormone for energy and warmth, thus adding to the imbalance caused by the increasing thyroid needs of the pregnancy itself. Patients fall behind on their thyroid reserves, don't produce enough progesterone, and miscarry.

Since thyroid needs advance along with pregnancy, seasonal upward adjustments that were made in the fall need to be increased further, whereas in the spring, when I usually decrease doses, I would tend to keep the dose the same.

Take Action

If you conceive during the summer, have your thyroid status reevaluated as autumn approaches, and consider an increase in dose. This is prudent practice for any woman, but especially important for those with preexisting hypothyroidism. Pregnancy "symptoms" such as fatigue and acid reflux may indicate thyroid depletion and the need for dosage reevaluation. My patient Ruth put it well: "God knows I would have been equally grateful with fatigue and morning sickness, but I haven't had one day of problems, whether it's the T3 or taking good care of myself, or both."

GET ADEQUATE THYROID TREATMENT THROUGHOUT PREGNANCY

Many women feel that if they make it past the first trimester, they're home free. Unfortunately, this is not the case with hypothyroidism.

Second-trimester risks. While second-trimester miscarriages are relatively rare, they appear to be more common in hypothyroidism. A study in the *British Medical Journal's Journal of Medical Screening* (1999) showed that the chances of miscarriage in the second trimester (weeks 12–24) are four times higher among women with hypothyroidism. The findings reveal that women with hypothyroidism during pregnancy have a 3.8 percent risk for late miscarriage as opposed to women with normal thyroid function, who only have a 0.9 percent rate. In this study, six out of every one hundred late miscarriages could be attributed to thyroid deficiency during pregnancy.

Third-trimester risks. Women with untreated hypothyroidism near the time of delivery are in danger of high blood pressure and premature delivery. High blood pressure is especially dangerous in late-stage pregnancy. Also called preeclampsia or toxemia, high blood pressure during pregnancy is more common in a woman's first pregnancy. The first signs may be weight gain of five to ten pounds within a week, as a result of fluid retention. Headaches and blurred vision may also occur.

Though preeclampsia can occur at any time during a woman's pregnancy, women with hypothyroidism are at higher risk near term. Fetal complications of preeclampsia include inadequate fetal growth, premature labor, and fetal distress during delivery.

Take Action

Physiologic doses of T4 and T3 are critical to provide the thyroid reserve needed to carry a pregnancy to term. During pregnancy, the physiologic need is higher. In addition, as Ruth's success with natural thyroid extract demonstrates, women who do not respond to synthetic hormones may also need the "other" natural thyroid hormones that are not available in synthetic form.

At the first signs of symptoms—excessive swelling—contact your doctor. He or she may recommend bed rest, or even hospitalization if your problem is severe. By no means reduce your salt intake, as some health sources suggest for swelling, as this has negative consequences not only on your developing child but on your thyroid health.

Dosing Guidelines During Pregnancy

Thyroid dosing needs may increase during pregnancy, so I monitor closely for symptoms and seasonal requirements (as discussed above). With proper adjustments, patients who developed fatigue or acid reflux will be amazed by how much better they feel a week or two after the dose increases.

Adjustments in dosage are usually made with T4; dye-free T4 is available in 50-mcg increments, making it easy to add or subtract one or two tablets a week. The slight changes up or down usually have little effect on the physiologic ratio, so there's usually no need to change T3 doses.

At the time of delivery, thyroid requirements decrease significantly for the mother, so I generally advise no thyroid treatment at all for the typical one- or two-day hospital stay. During summer months of delivery, my patients generally resume taking thyroid medication at about 80 to 85 percent of their prior dose. If the delivery happens in the winter, I typically leave the doses unchanged; the seasonal change offsets the reduced postpartum need.

THE EFFECTS ON INFANTS OF MATERNAL HYPOTHYROIDISM

Hypothyroidism in infants is generally not caused by inadequate maternal thyroid levels late in pregnancy. The fetal thyroid develops early in pregnancy, and the placenta isolates the fetus. However, transient newborn hypothyroidism can occur as a result of antibodies transferred from the mother, iodine deficiency, and other problems. Quick treatment of the newborn with adequate T4 is crucial to early mental development.

A highly publicized report estimated that untreated infants could lose up to three to five IQ points per month during the first year. Immediate treatment with thyroid hormone can minimize the harm. But according to a 1999 Canadian study, in spite of early treatment, learning disabilities were evident in the third grade (ages nine to ten) in many children who had received early treatment. And problems with memory, attention, and spatial processing continued into adolescence.

A more recent investigation yields some disturbing news. The study showed that birth defects are more common in the offspring of untreated hypothyroid women. Results of the study, presented at the 2002 annual meeting of the Society for Maternal-Fetal Medicine, showed that babies born to women with overactive or underactive thyroid also were at increased risk of a variety of anomalies, including cleft lip or palate and extra fingers. In addition, infants born to women with hypothyroidism were more prone to cardiac problems even if the mothers were medicated.

These studies emphasize the importance for mothers to maintain *healthy* thyroid hormone balances during pregnancy.

Take Action

Make sure that your doctor is monitoring your thyroid levels closely, every twelve weeks minimum. Keep attuned to symptoms of hypothyroidism that are easily confused with pregnancy: fatigue, acid reflux, mental fogginess. Any dramatic change in your symptoms should be immediately communicated to your doctor.

AFTER YOU GIVE BIRTH . . .

Known as postpartum thyroiditis, hypothyroidism surfaces in 5 to 10 percent of women within a year of delivery. And women with diabetes are three times more likely to develop postpartum thyroiditis.

Postpartum thyroiditis often occurs when thyroid autoantibodies are high during the pregnancy, causing thyroid inflammation (thyroiditis) after delivery. If you tested positive for TPO-Ab early in pregnancy, your chances of developing postpartum thyroiditis are as high as 50 percent.

Although postpartum thyroiditis may disappear on its own after a year or less, the AACE estimates that 50 percent will develop permanent hypothyroidism within five years of diagnosis.

Symptoms of Postpartum Thyroiditis

Postpartum thyroiditis follows a pattern similar to that of autoimmune thyroiditis: A period of hyperthyroidism is usually followed by hypothyroidism. The *hyper*thyroid phase can begin anywhere from the first to the sixth month of pregnancy and lasts up to two months. Symptoms are usually mild compared to Graves' disease: Palpitations, weight loss, heat intolerance, irritability, and fatigue are most common.

The *hypo*thyroid phase develops about four to eight months after delivery and can last four months or longer. Notable symptoms are muscle and joint pain, tiredness, loss of concentration, and constipation. The hallmark symptom, however, is depression, which is difficult to distinguish from postpartum depression. Again, the AACE reports that about 20 percent of new mothers have the baby blues, and a significant percentage have some form of depression.

How to Handle Postpartum Thyroiditis

Treatment of postpartum thyroiditis depends on the stage and severity. In mild cases, I might take a "wait and see" approach, with hopes that the symptoms will disappear. If they are very bothersome, I'd treat *hyper*thyroid symptoms to help the patient feel more comfortable. For example, I might prescribe beta-adrenergic blockers to slow heart palpitations or a sedative to calm nerves.

Hypothyroidism that's interfering with daily life can be treated with hormone replacement therapy—assuming you're not already taking it. Return to your doctor after a year and revisit your symptoms and thyroid status. If you still feel hypothyroid, you may need to initiate thyroid hormone therapy.

Breast-Feeding Concerns with Thyroid Replacement

If you are taking the proper dosage, thyroid replacement hormone poses little to no risk to your baby. However, if you become hyperthyroid, you may pass on too much thyroid medicine to the baby. But this is rarely a clinical problem, since the extra thyroid hormone transferred will suppress the infant's TSH, reducing his own thyroid hormone production to maintain a proper balance. Your doctor should monitor your thyroid hormones closely to make sure that you are within the right range for you.

Some hypothyroid mothers have problems producing enough milk. A lactation consultant may help, or you may need to supplement with formula—but not soy, which is goitrogenic. If your baby has lactose allergies, discuss other options such as goat milk with your pediatrician, or consult the La Leche League.

Will My Baby Inherit My Thyroid Problem?

The chance of passing on a specific gene for hypothyroidism is very low. But both hypothyroidism and autoimmunity tend to run in families, so your child is predisposed to thyroid deficiencies that may not show up until she is in her twenties or thirties. Early signs of evolving thyroid deficiency show up as cognitive (learning) difficulties in children (chapter 9) and in teenagers (chapter 10) when they experience PMS and other symptoms.

——— •◆• ———

Giving Your Child the Best Start in Infancy and Childhood

A caveat: In the following pages you'll read some facts about congenital hypothyroidism that might concern you. When hypothyroidism is caught and treated early in infancy, the vast majority of children have absolutely no problems with mental or physical development. So please take the following information as it was intended: to give you guidelines—and reasons—for speaking with your doctor about treating hypothyroidism in infants.

METABOLIC PROFILE

Within the first few minutes of birth, fast and furious metabolic changes happen. During delivery and immediately after the umbilical cord is cut, newborns experience an intense surge in TSH. This helps them to generate the energy and heat needed to adjust to the rapid change in temperature from the uterus to the outside environment. As we'll see later in this chapter, the adaptation and growth process in infants creates an exceptional demand for thyroid hormone, which must be in place during gestation, in the womb. If not, as noted in the preceding chapter, a very serious thyroid deficiency may occur called congenital hypothyroidism.

CONGENITAL HYPOTHYROIDISM

If you have just learned that your baby has congenital hypothyroidism, you are probably very concerned. In this short chapter, I hope to share basic information and resources to help deepen your understanding about the causes, risks, and treatments available for your child now and in the future. I refer you to the Resources section at the back of this book for sources of more information about this troubling condition.

Congenital hypothyroidism is defined as the loss of thyroid hormone that affects newborns ("congenital"). In most cases, congenital hypothyroidism results from improper development of the thyroid gland. But it can occur when the gland is absent or in the wrong location. The result is insufficient amounts of thyroid hormone. In the maturing infant, lack of thyroid hormone has serious developmental consequences, such as slow growth and reduced mental function—a syndrome called cretinism.

Cardiac and other abnormalities can occur with congenital hypothyroidism, but they're more common in infants who are born early.

A Rare, Often-Unexplained Condition

About one out of every four thousand white infants is born with congenital hypothyroidism, but as with the general population, the incidence is much lower among African American children—one out of every thirteen thousand. There is no uniform cause for this abnormality. Rarely, children acquire a genetic (inherited) form of hypothyroidism, although a recent study suggests a genetic link between thyroid abnormalities in symptom-free family members and infants.

In some children, the symptoms (see below) are only temporary, and when parents and doctors are certain that it has not recurred (usually by age three), medication can be discontinued. But in cases of true congenital hypothyroidism, children must remain on thyroid replacement therapy for their entire lives.

One study of a baby born with hemangiomas, an abnormal proliferation of blood vessels, showed that these hemangiomas might cause hypothyroidism. The hemangiomas seem to have a type of deiodinase enzyme that inactivates T4 in the blood. Hypothyroidism results if the thyroid fails to keep pace with the degraded T4. Since hemangiomas are present in 5 to 10 percent of one-year-olds, this may be a common cause of hypothyroidism and should be investigated by your baby's pediatrician.

Testing Is Not Always Straightforward

Most hospitals routinely draw blood from the infant's heel (a "heel stick" sample) for a panel of tests that often includes testing for TSH level. If the mother was hypothyroid during pregnancy, or there is a family history of hypothyroidism, then you should make sure that a TSH test is included on the panel. But keep in mind that the results obtained within the first twenty-four hours of life may be misleading.

Due to the swell of thyroid hormones in the first minutes after delivery, an initial screening that's performed in the first twenty-four hours of life, as is common, would yield falsely high TSH levels—a false positive for hypothyroidism. The baby's circulating TSH concentration may be higher than normal (normal infant levels are less than 20 mU/l in most laboratories). So levels of 20 to 50 mU/l in the first twenty-four hours of life may reflect nothing more than this neonatal TSH surge and not congenital hypothyroidism, particularly if the total thyroid hormone concentration (T4) is normal.

In a study of 122,000 infants, congenital hypothyroidism was most likely if the initial TSH was greater than 60 mU/l, with 45 to 60 mU/l being a vague zone. In states that have initiated mandatory second screening at ten to fourteen days of life, this unusual pattern disappears, since the early TSH surge diminishes by the *third day of life*. Any newborn suspected of having true primary congenital hypothyroidism should have a complete thyroid profile within the first two to three weeks of life.

In some cases, hypothyroidism does not make itself evident until after the heel-stick test is performed—more reason for careful monitoring of infant symptoms.

If your baby's doctor suspects hypothyroidism, he or she may also take an X ray of the legs to look at the ends of the bones. In babies with hypothyroidism, the bones are not mature. A thyroid scan should be done to determine the location or absence of the thyroid gland. These tests—bone age and thyroid scan—can be done at the time of diagnosis.

Symptoms of Congenital Hypothyroidism

Babies will often seem perfectly normal at birth. And when present, the symptoms of hypothyroidism are not very specific—lots of newborns have similar characteristics without hypothyroidism. Indeed, the "classic" symptoms of congenital hypothyroidism actually occur in only some infants:

- Increased birth weight
- Large, despite having poor feeding habits
- Puffy face, swollen tongue
- Hoarse cry
- Low muscle tone
- Cold extremities
- Persistent constipation, bloated or full to the touch
- Lack of energy, sleeps most of the time, appears tired even when awake
- Little to no growth
- Poor feeding due to decreased appetite
- Prolonged jaundice (yellow skin)

These symptoms should be confirmed by screening at birth and after the initial birth surge to identify hypothyroidism.

Treatment of Congenital Hypothyroidism

As with adults, thyroid hormone supplies the metabolic power for all body organs to function normally. This is especially important in the developing infant, where it is not just a case of feeling well enough to function, but to function at all. Physical, emotional, and mental growth hinges on adequate thyroid hormone.

Thyroid hormone is available as a pill. Usually, infants are given synthetic T4. Again, the purest form available with the least dyes and excipients is the 50-mcg tablet. The starting dose is between 25 and 50 mcg per day. Usually, the pill is crushed and added to water, formula, or breast milk. The dose will be adjusted based on blood tests.

Most infants fare very well with close monitoring and treatment of hypothyroidism. But some children may experience developmental problems later in life. It is especially important to keep a close watch on children as they grow, to ensure that they are receiving the proper dose of hormone.

You can expect your doctor to set up a schedule of visits every three months or so to ensure adequate blood levels of thyroid hormone. To give your baby the best chance of healthy mental and physical development, a lifelong regimen of daily medication is critical.

CHILDHOOD HYPOTHYROIDISM

Mood swings, weight gain, fatigue, and daydreamy behavior in school—these are some of the vague symptoms that can first warn of hypothyroidism in children. Other more typically hypothyroid symptoms may come about slowly and without much warning: a goiter (swelling at the bottom of the neck near the collarbone), cold intolerance, dry skin, puffiness, decreased appetite, behavioral and learning problems (mostly related to fatigue and brain fog), and even dyslexia (particularly among boys). Your child may suddenly stop growing as fast as he was before, or her teeth seem to come in later than her peers' teeth do.

One mother described how her eight-year-old girl was so dreamy in class that she missed large parts of her lessons—and her grades reflected it. Another parent said, "The biggest thing I see is fatigue and emotional immaturity. Everything is a crisis—it's like she's got PMS, but she's only seven! We're always walking on eggshells around her."

A still different scenario was reported by a mother whose six-year-old son had kept up fine on the growth charts until he hit the age of four. Today he weighs only forty-five pounds and is still wearing 4/5 clothes. His TSH levels were slightly above normal at 6.5, and he was positive for thyroid autoantibodies, yet his pediatrician refused treatment, claiming that autoimmune disease is "overblown."

None of these children had hypothyroidism as infants (congenital hypothyroidism); they have what is called acquired hypothyroidism, which is hypothyroidism that arises after the age of two. But some have a family history of thyroid disease—that is, a direct relative who is known to have had some sort of thyroid problem. And in all cases, the parent fundamentally, intuitively knew that something was wrong.

Follow Your Instincts

Having a gut feeling that even subtle symptoms are not normal for your child is probably one of the best indicators of the need for further investigation. Unfortunately, as is the case with adults, hypothyroidism does not always fit into neat diagnostic packages. And it often takes the persistence of a parent/caregiver advocate to find a doctor who will test, and if the test results are in or near the normal range, to treat. Being a strong advocate begins with acquiring a solid knowledge base. Start here.

The ABC's of Childhood Hypothyroidism

A Is for Abnormal Growth

Like the case described above, your child may be growing fine for a year or two, but suddenly his growth pattern changes *for him.* This doesn't always mean that your child is shorter than other children—it means that he's not growing at the same *rate* that he was before. He could actually be taller than his classmates if he was well above average at one point. Take this drop-off in growth as a sign that something might be amiss, particularly if thyroid problems or autoimmune problems run in your family.

B Is for Behavioral and Learning Problems

There is some evidence that children of mothers with inadequately treated hypothyroidism could show later-stage learning and behavioral problems. Though the risk is small, and the evidence is not conclusive, parents would be wise to keep their eye on their child's development.

In acquired (noncongenital) hypothyroidism, learning and behavioral issues seem to have a different timbre. Recent research shows that dyslexia may be a problem in children with Hashimoto's thyroiditis. Problems associated with dyslexia include poor speech development, spelling, and handwriting. Children may also confuse their left from their right, and reverse letters or numbers. Keep in mind that all of these problems are very common in children who are just learning to read and write. Concerns should be acted on if these problems become a persistent pattern that causes your child to lag behind in school in spite of high intelligence.

Children with Hashimoto's may also exhibit problems in concentrating, and they may have problems with reading and attention. Poor school performance in spite of high intelligence suggests an underlying problem that may be traced to hypothyroidism. Hashimoto's should be considered, especially if there is a family history of autoimmune disease.

As new treatments for attention deficit disorder (ADD) become available, publicity about this condition floods parenting magazines and the general press. Because ADD and ADHD (ADD with hyperactivity) are much more top-of-mind than hypothyroidism, and symptoms can overlap, there is some danger that your child may be misdiagnosed as having ADD, leading to treatment with methylphenidate (Ritalin) and other drugs that may significantly and unnecessarily compromise your child's quality of life.

Most people think of ADD children as being "hyper," but according to the Attention Deficit Disorder Association, "Individuals with ADD *without hyperactivity* [emphasis in original] are sometimes thought of as daydreamers or 'absent-minded professors.' The non-hyperactive children with ADD most often seem to be girls (though girls can have ADD with hyperactivity, and boys can have ADD without hyperactivity)."

Psychiatrists use the *Diagnostics Standards Manual—IV* (fourth edition) to diagnose attention-deficit disorder. ADD is highly suspected if children have six out of the nine symptoms below for six months or longer.

- Often fails to give close attention to details or makes careless mistakes in schoolwork, work, or other activities.
- Often has difficulty in sustaining attention in tasks or play activities.
- Often does not seem to listen when spoken to directly.
- Often does not follow through on instructions and fails to finish schoolwork, chores, or duties in the workplace (not due to oppositional behavior or doesn't understand instructions).
- Often has difficulty organizing tasks and activities.
- Often avoids, dislikes, or is reluctant to engage in tasks or activities that require sustained mental effort (such as schoolwork or homework).
- Often loses things necessary for tasks or activities (e.g., toys, school assignments, pencils, books, tools).
- Often easily distracted by extraneous stimuli.
- Often forgetful in daily activities.

If your child has six of these nine symptoms, he or she could be diagnosed as having ADD. But there is great danger in jumping to this conclusion. It is easy to see how the fatigue typical of hypothyroidism can result in many of these symptoms as well. For children with a family history of hypothyroidism and other signs of this disorder, *there is little harm in a diagnostic trial of thyroid medication.* In addition to close communication with your physician, work with your child's teacher to establish a way of documenting your child's progress with your medication (see below for my recommendations for starting doses).

The basic hypothyroid symptoms are similar to those for adults, with some child-specific additions. And as with adults, they progress slowly and may accumulate over time: fatigue, weight gain, reduced appetite, constipation, cold intolerance, dry skin, and delayed sexual development.

C Is for Rare Clinical Causes of Hypothyroidism

These include diseases of the pituitary, hypothalamus, and tumors or cysts between these two glands.

D Is for My Two-Week Diagnostic Trial

If signs and symptoms point strongly toward hypothyroidism, even when test results don't, there is no harm in a diagnostic trial. The ultimate answer to the question of whether a child should be on thyroid hormone is the same as it is with adults. For me, improvement with thyroid replacement after a long pattern of bothersome problems, not a laboratory result, establishes the fundamental diagnosis.

My recommendation is to start young patients on 50 mcg T4 at one-half tablet daily and instruct them to report responses as they occur. If the child appears to have a fast response and *hyper*thyroid symptoms, such as palpitations, I have them stop T4 for a few days and then restart at a lower dose—for example, one-half of one 50-mcg tablet on Mondays, Wednesdays, and Fridays. Once the tolerated dose of T4 is found, I would give 98 percent T4 and 2 percent T3.

Again, my 2 percent solution—98 percent T4 and 2 percent T3—applies to children as it does to adults. This approach should provide enough hormones for normal metabolic development and growth. Talk to your child's doctor about these recommendations.

E Is for Establishing a Lifelong Foundation

Unlike congenital hypothyroidism, treatment is not as urgent in children with acquired disease, but it is essential to take positive action and to develop a plan. Children are establishing a foundation for lifelong confidence, developing their sense of selves, and neurologically peaking in their ability to acquire and process new information. If not treated early, short stature can be permanent. A misdiagnosis at this time could rob children of their childhood—and stigmatize them for life.

F Is for Follow-Through

If your child's hypothyroidism is affecting his or her academic performance or behavior, it might be helpful to work with your child's school—a team of professionals who understand your child's problem and who, with you, can pinpoint skill areas where the child may need improvement. It is important to remember that hypothyroidism is usually a chronic disorder, and continued, long-term support may be necessary.

Arrange a meeting with your child's school team as soon as your child is diagnosed. The team may include teacher(s), principal, school psychologist or counselor, and school nurse. You are the central focus of the team. Prepare to become "case manager and advocate" for your child. This means that you will help coordinate the efforts of your child's health care team (pediatrician and/or pediatric endocrinologist) and education team—and continue your own research into hypothyroidism.

Keeping Up with Your Kids As They Change

The child's constant growth puts an exceptionally high demand on metabolic and hormonal systems, and what works today may not work in three or four months or a year. Here's how you can keep up:

- Engage a pediatric endocrinologist.
- Keep a close eye on symptoms as a warning sign that dosage may need to be adjusted.
- Make sure that blood levels of TSH and T4 are monitored routinely. Like adults, your child's "personal best" test result may be higher or lower than the norm. It is part of the treatment challenge to find the level at which your child feels best and to continually monitor symptoms and test results to gauge dosage.
- If your child is old enough, involve her in the treatment by teaching her about the importance of a dosage routine. Educate her about how to take her medication (at the same time each day with regard to food and vitamins).
- Give your child extra support and confidence. When something is wrong, even young children are apt to blame themselves. Let your child know that he is not responsible for his condition and that with medicine and good nutrition, he can overcome many of the symptoms. With chronic illness of any sort, children need to be reminded all the more that your love is there in sickness and in health.

- Get support. Contact local hypothyroid organizations to meet parents of other hypothyroid children—or form one yourself by putting up a bulletin in your pediatric endocrinologist's office. Perhaps your doctor will agree to host meetings and give informal discussions about issues relating to childhood hypothyroidism.
- Many on-line support groups are available for parents, particularly the support groups at About.com, Yahoo.com, and the Magic Foundation. See Resources at the back of this book.

Chapter 10

Balancing on the Edge:
Adolescence and PMS

It all started when I was thirteen. I had severe migraines; I was exhausted, nauseous, and had terrible PMS. I missed forty days of school my eighth-grade year, and I had no social life. Basically, I was a mess. Over the next two years I saw allergists, neurologists, and endocrinologists. The allergists said I was allergic to dust, but the treatment didn't help. The first endocrinologist said my thyroid tests (TSH) were normal and there was nothing wrong except that my hormones were out of whack because of puberty. Finally, I found Dr. Blanchard in 2001, who said I have hypothyroidism. He gave me thyroid treatments and said it would take a while, but actually my tiredness and nausea stopped within a few weeks. Now everything's great. I have my friends and my life back. My story opened the door for other people in my family to realize that they might be hypothyroid, too.

—Nancy R., aged sixteen

I link Nancy's case and teenage issues in this chapter with PMS because so many menstrual and reproductive problems begin with a misdiagnosis in adolescence. Nancy was admitted to the hospital twice because of severe headaches and had every test under the sun. When she first came in, she was a sullen person being dragged in by her mother. Since starting treatment, I don't think she'd had a single headache. She's a super student and active on the track team. Today she comes in with her mother like they're best girlfriends.

Nancy's case is typical of many histories I hear from women in their forties. They have a teenage history of coldness, or being so tired after school that they need a nap. They sleep till noon on weekends and have two or three periods a year. They go away to college and miss their periods for nine months. The gynecologist puts them on the birth control pill to "regulate their periods." This further shakes up a young woman's thyroid hormone balance: Estrogen increases the amount of "bound" thyroid hormone, leaving less free, active hormone to do the job.

How many times have I heard from these women in their forties—many of whom were infertile, many divorced, not interested in sex, so depressed they have just enough energy to sit around—that their problems started in adolescence? And then I treat them—again in the face of a normal TSH—and they tell me that at forty-two they feel the best they have in their entire lives and that they finally, finally have regular periods without being regulated by oral contraceptives.

To believe my patients, which I do completely, is to understand that detecting and treating symptoms of hypothyroidism in adolescence is the key to avoiding a lifetime of misery.

HYPOTHYROIDISM IN ADOLESCENCE

Adolescence is a time of explosive mental and physical growth—a time when the demands for thyroid hormone are great. If natural hormonal levels can't keep pace with these demands, the patient suffers in many ways. That's why, especially in cases where there's a family history of thyroid disease of any kind, or of autoimmune disease, you should think thyroid when your son or daughter shows symptoms.

Puberty is also a time when the female hormone estrogen is on the rise for women. As mentioned, the estrogen link is being investigated as a factor for autoimmune diseases, which primarily strike women—and do so during their reproductive years.

Diagnosis Is a Challenge

When the body's in constant flux, as it is during adolescence, it's hard to get a fix on what's normal and what's not. In addition to the classic symptoms that characterize hypothyroidism, the following symptoms may dominate:

- Fatigue
- Short stature
- Delayed or premature puberty
- Depression
- Goiter (swollen thyroid gland)
- Menstrual abnormalities

Fatigue

Because adolescence marks such dramatic physical and emotional change, it's hard for teens and their parents to know what's normal and what's not. Many of the symptoms of hypothyroidism are typical of teenage years. It is easy to pass off fatigue as a sign of adolescence—because it is! More than 40 percent of healthy teenagers say that they feel tired, and it is often reflected in their ability to sleep longer than most adults would think humanly possible.

It is normal for anyone to feel tired after exerting effort. And to feel replenished by rest. It is *not* normal if your child is sleepy during the day, has insomnia and irritability, aches, headaches, and decreased appetite. This fatigue can take its toll on attention span and learning capacities, translating into poor grades, objectionable behavior at school, and misdiagnosis as ADD (see pages 141–143). It can also take an emotional toll. Untreated patients who struggle with fatigue or brain fog can be labeled lazy or sluggish, causing significant mental anguish.

As a forty-three-year-old patient commented: "I had stopped growing and had late puberty. It was agonizing—I felt like I was abnormal, not like the other girls. It undermined my confidence and sense of self—something I still experience sometimes to this day." *Any*thing that makes teens feel different or weird is cause for dire pain. And hypothyroidism causes many differences.

Growth Rate

Thyroid disease may slow down or interfere with your child's normal physical development. As a gauge for what's normal, look at your own family: When did you go through puberty? At what age did you have your first period? Develop facial and genital hair? This is a fairly good indicator of when your child will do the same, but it is certainly *not* an absolute. Hypothyroidism may be suspected, however, if there are significant lags in the *rate of growth*. The time of the teenage "growth spurt" differs from one child to the next, and your child's peers should not be the measure of normalcy. If you have any concerns about your child's growth rate, especially if he or she suffers other symptoms and there's a family history of thyroid problems, I would definitely encourage a thyroid investigation.

Puberty

Delayed puberty is a suggestive sign of hypothyroidism. Adolescents may appear three or four years younger than they actually are. *Premature* puberty may also occur, whereby children exhibit signs of puberty at an early age, before age eleven. Either of these conditions should prompt a visit to your child's doctor.

Depression

Mood swings are a hallmark of adolescence, and depression is very common. Mild depression occurs in up to 10 percent of high school students, moderate depression in 5 to 6 percent, and major depression in 1 to 2 percent. If *you* were depressed as a teen, your child might experience depression at around the same age. Depression should be taken seriously if it persists longer than two weeks and is not caused by any specific event: More than half of adolescent suicidal behaviors stem from depression. Consider depression as a source of problems if your child withdraws, starts doing poorly in school, self-medicates by substance abuse, or starts exhibiting behavioral problems. Younger adolescents may be less able to explain inner feelings or moods, whereas adolescents in their midteens may believe that to do so is a sign of "weakness." Depression in adolescence is overlooked at least as often as in other age groups.

When is depression an offshoot of hypothyroidism? Again, investigation into your child's thyroid status should be top-of-mind if depression occurs along with other hypothyroid symptoms and if there's a family history of thyroid/autoimmune disease. In my practice, this scenario would be enough justification for a Two-Week Diagnostic Trial of hormone replacement. A positive response to my trial regimen (as outlined in chapter 4) should provide good evidence of hypothyroidism and is much safer and faster than antidepressant medication.

Goiters

A *goiter* may appear in girls as their estrogen levels increase, just before they begin to menstruate. A checkup is vital if you think your child has any swelling at the bottom of her neck—it may be indicative of a thyroid nodule. Though most nodules are harmless, in children they can occasionally be cancerous.

Menstrual Abnormalities

Menstruation usually begins after the age of nine and before the age of sixteen. Hypothyroidism in adolescence is most commonly associated with delayed puberty and sometimes decreased stature (height). Rarely, hypothyroidism in childhood is associated with precocious puberty with enlargement of the pituitary gland and other pituitary abnormalities such as excessive production of a hormone called prolactin. These possibilities should be considered *before* treatment with thyroid medication.

Irregular or scant periods, as well as extraordinarily heavy menstruation, are other traits of hypothyroidism problems that start with puberty and set the stage for infertility and other problems throughout a woman's reproductive life. Since menstrual abnormalities are common in the first year of puberty, it's important to keep a close eye on symptoms before rushing in for diagnosis. I would not prescribe thyroid replacement unless problems continue for longer than one year.

PREMENSTRUAL SYNDROME

The link between PMS and hypothyroidism was a turning point in my practice. My unorthodox treatment approach began with a PMS patient in the mid-1980s. It was around this time that the subject enjoyed a brief spotlight in the medical literature.

In 1986, N.D. Brayshaw and D.D. Brayshaw published a letter in the *New England Journal of Medicine* announcing that thirty-four out of thirty-four women with premenstrual syndrome had experienced a remarkable improvement in symptoms with thyroid hormone. For reasons not explained by the authors, their drug protocol was 25 mcg T4 (the smallest available commercial dose) that was increased by 25 mcg each month. The dramatic improvements in the first month of therapy prompted them to rush to print with a letter to the editor—and they were never heard from again! Although their work was discredited—including anecdotal reports of side effects; no surprise with the consistent climb in dosage—the initial results intrigued me.

The Brayshaws' letter prompted two groups of academicians to set up formal studies. In 1990, a report published by the Marshfield Clinic, a respected medical center in Wisconsin, compared the responses of PMS patients to three treatment regimens: placebo, T4 based on patient weight, and 95 mcg T4. The two T4 regimens had no better effect on PMS than placebo.

In 1993, a group at the National Institutes of Health enrolled thirty PMS patients on a seven-month double-blind, placebo-controlled crossover trial—the best design in the industry. In this study, patients took either T4 (100 mcg) or a placebo for three months. After a period of "rest" in between treatments, the subject groups switched for three months. The placebo group switched to T4, and the T4 patients switched to placebo. Neither group knew whether they were taking placebo or T4. This study concluded flatly that T4 was not effective in PMS, though the researchers acknowledged that some patients might have a slight thyroid defect and require hormone.

It's no wonder that hypothyroidism has been wholly dismissed as a cause of PMS. Indeed, in a recent review of the premenstrual syndrome, thyroid hormone was not even mentioned. But one issue plagued me . . .

More Isn't Better: Finding the Physiologic Dose

Why did T4 bring initial success in the Brayshaw study, while it failed so completely in the two academic studies? The main difference was dosage. The Brayshaws started with a low T4 dose, whereas the other studies used four times the amount. But why did a lower dose succeed where a higher dose failed?

This question planted the seed for a theory that has guided my success in patients with a wide range of hypothyroid symptoms: Thyroid supplementation must be physiologic, not pharmacologic. The corollaries of this approach are that the dose must reflect the body's needs (the 2 percent T3 solution), and more is not better.

Indeed, early on I had the same experience in my clinical practice as my published colleagues. Patients would feel great for two to three months on T4, then come back to me reporting that their response had faded. The temptation was to increase the T4 dose, but inevitably, this would result in a recurrence of PMS *plus* increased fatigue and weight gain. TSH results would be in the lower end of normal, technically indicating excessive dosage. However, when I institute low T4 doses (about 25 mcg) with 2 percent T3, patients experience dramatic improvements, which persist unless other factors require a reevaluation of dose, such as seasonal changes, pregnancy, or menopause.

The proof is in the TSH result. Even though a patient is receiving T4 and T3, TSH results do not fall into the *hyper*thyroid range. Sometimes they even *rise* on thyroid treatment. This pattern flies in the face of conventional medical philosophy, which asserts that adding thyroid hormone will produce a reduction in TSH levels. (Remember the lessons from chapter 3: TSH levels reflect a lack of thyroid hormone; they increase when levels are low and decrease when thyroid hormone levels are high.)

My explanation is that PMS patients experience an extreme overstimulation of deiodinase enzyme in the pituitary, leading to excessive local generation of T3 and false suppression of TSH. In essence, the pituitary is flooded with T3 and blinded to the need for thyroid hormone, so it fails to send out signals for TSH to be produced. The aim of treatment must be to normalize pituitary proportions of T4 and T3. Giving too much T4 will just aggravate the problem. Slowly, slowly, patients must be given physiologic doses of T4 and T3 (i.e., 25 mcg T4 and 0.5 mcg T3). Over time, the pituitary proportions will normalize, but it may take up to one year. Patience has its virtues and its physical rewards. In many cases, however, patients have very rapid, very gratifying responses.

Chapter 11

It's Also a Guy Thing

When John came to me in February 2001 at the age of forty-two, he was reluctant to open up at first. "I know enough about health to be dangerous, but not enough to be effective, so I diagnosed myself with lupus, multiple sclerosis, anything else. I was hesitant to tell Dr. Blanchard all my symptoms because I thought I was losing my mind."

Upon questioning, I learned that John's problem traced back to his college years when he noted fatigue and was diagnosed with a goiter. He was never treated because his tests were normal. He described himself during his twenties as being hyper—always on the go, the life of the party, always doing something.

This scenario is typical of autoimmune thyroiditis. As the autoantibodies attack the thyroid, the thyroid becomes stimulated and reacts by sending out more hormone, so patients often report feeling hyper. But as thyroid function continues to diminish, hormone levels decrease and the opposite symptoms of hypothyroidism begin to surface.

By his mid- to late thirties, John's health had started to decline. "I was losing myself. I'd put on weight; I was falling asleep at my desk. The carpal tunnel was unmanageable—I was having numbness and tingling in my hands and feet—and became famous for my one-line e-mails, the pain was so bad. I started paranoically thinking that something desperate was wrong and went to a neurologist who said, 'No, you don't have MS.'"

But the worst, according to John, were the changes in his personality—the sense of losing the "color" in his life. And when I mentioned loss of libido along with other symptoms, he was relieved that I understood.

At the age of thirty-seven, John's TSH levels registered above normal. At this point, he began taking Synthroid. He was also taking Paxil, which helped somewhat with his depression. But with the triple-whammy of hypothyroidism (which slows testicular function), depression, and antidepressants, John's sex drive suffered to the point of being nonexistent. By the time he came to see me, his TSH (5.2) would be considered normal by some, but I knew otherwise.

Noting that he had allergy problems, I started John on 50 mcg Levothroid a day (a dye-free dose) at seventeen tablets per week, and 1.5 mcg T3 daily. His improvement was remarkable. As the season begins to change, John is on schedule for a dosage adjustment—he's starting to feel the symptoms of depression and carpal tunnel rear their heads.

According to John: "I went on T3 and I felt the difference within three weeks. I told my wife, 'I feel my personality coming back, my sense of humor coming back.' It really is a new day now."

As a male with hypothyroidism, John was aware of the female bias among doctors. It's true that women are up to ten times more likely to be hypothyroid. But one wonders whether more men would be diagnosed if men *and* their doctors were more aware of the signs and symptoms. It should be noted, too, that although the risk of primary hypothyroidism is much higher in women, thyroid nodules in men are 50 percent more likely to be cancerous. So it's vitally important to perform a neck check if you have symptoms of hypothyroidism (see page 27).

I keep repeating this statement, but it's worth it if it's the only fact that inspires you to seek treatment, and your doctor to actually test and treat you for hypothyroidism: Your risk increases for hypothyroidism if there's a family history of thyroid problems or autoimmune diseases (like rheumatoid arthritis, type I diabetes, systemic lupus erythematosus; see page 99). By a family history, I mean a history of disease in either men or women in your family. So in spite of a normal TSH, a family history and symptoms of hypothyroidism should warrant at least a diagnostic trial using physiologic doses of T4 and T3.

ARE MALE SYMPTOMS DIFFERENT FROM WOMEN'S?

Many of the symptoms may be the same—see chapter 1—but men may be more aware that their muscles seem larger, although they are not stronger. In addition, some men might be more sensitive to loss of libido and certainly to difficulties in getting an erection. Indeed, the thyroid was once considered a sex gland, and in lower mammals, it is directly connected to sexual organs. But in its role as "the great catalyst of energy" (to quote Louis Berman), the thyroid affects all body functions. When thyroid levels are low, everything slows down, including testicular function.

Men may also be more prone to other related problems, such as stress and infection. Having read up on the subject,

John wonders whether his hypothyroidism was associated with the stress of quitting smoking or the bout he had with mononucleosis, both of which happened around the time of his diagnosis.

Younger men are at a greatly increased risk of heart disease than women. Left untreated, hypothyrodism further elevates the chances of heart disease by raising cholesterol levels and by contributing to weight gain and insulin resistance. Men also may be more sensitive to hair loss, though it can be at least equally traumatic when it happens to women. Unlike typical "male pattern balding," hypothyroidism causes hair to thin all over the scalp—and other parts of the body—due to slower cellular turnover.

Gaining weight and difficulty in losing it is a universal complaint among both women and men, and men will benefit from my diet plan (see chapter 16) as much as women.

MORE YOU CAN DO

In addition to making sure that your thyroid levels are in balance, you might want to consider these nutritional or alternative approaches:

- Add testosterone to help boost your libido and minimize certain types of hair loss. It's available by prescription as a patch or a gel. Ask your doctor about the form that might suit you best.
- Certain types of exercise help hypothyroid men lose weight. Alternating fast and slow running in one-minute intervals is more effective than running at a steady pace, according to a ten-week study that was reported in the journal *Medicine and Science in Sports and Exercise* in 2001.

- Check out other factors that may be contributing to loss of libido, such as other medications (antihypertension medicine, antidepressants). It's also important to rule out other conditions such as depression and diabetes, that can play a role in reduced sexual function.
- Get the support you need. You are not alone. If it helps, contact other men with hypothyroidism via local support groups or the Internet, such as the men's support group at Yahoo.com. A great place to pick up tips!

Chapter 12

Menopause: Finding Your Balance Amid Change

I was so tired of doctors classifying all my symptoms as menopausal! It started in my early forties, more than ten years ago, and so the doctor put me on a synthetic estrogen and I couldn't tolerate it—which is lucky considering what we now know about hormone replacement therapy. So I went to a female gynecologist, who recommended a hysterectomy. She was my age! I was depressed, I was tired, but at the age of forty-four, I refused to give in to old age or menopause. I went to a number of holistic people and ended up with one who gave me Dr. Blanchard's name. I had little faith. The questions he asked me were right on the money—they were all about symptoms I felt I'd have to deal with for the rest of my life, like the sleep disturbances. You know that tired, worn-out feeling—all those things that I think menopause can make you feel: that it's too late, that life has passed me by. And sexually, I was indifferent, just not there anymore. I just don't buy aging. I don't dress old, I don't feel old, I'm very active—but I was going that route. I simply wasn't fine with the idea that my life would just trudge on.

—Sherry R., aged fifty-six

When Sherry came to see me in 2001 at the age of fifty-five, she had very significant thinning of the outer eyebrows, slight enlargement on the right side of the thyroid gland, and slow reflexes. Her T4 was 5.7, and her TSH was 1.25—on the low end of normal. I began therapy with one-half tablet of 50 mcg Synthroid daily, and she demonstrated remarkable improvement in her symptoms in about ten days. At that time, I added 0.5 mcg of T3. She also received the estradiol patch, along with a cream combination of progesterone and testosterone.

Sherry's response to this therapy:

I never had a weight issue until menopause, and then my whole metabolism changed. With the T4 and T3, I didn't see any significant weight loss at first, but I'm certainly not putting on weight. I really need to exercise, and I don't! But my energy is way up, and I have a positive outlook. My daughter is in the front house, and I'm in the back with my granddaughter nearby. I think just having the energy to keep up with my grandchildren is another gift. I totally embrace it—I'm so excited about it!

It comes back to my attitude—a good attitude that carries over into everything. A year ago I let my hair grow long and it's been fun and I enjoy it. My friends don't even believe I'm as old as I am. Some of it's genetics, but mostly it's because I'm smiling and my attitude is positive and fun. And I bought a convertible. Every chance I get, I'm out in it!

Oh, yes. My sex life—it's been quite good! At one point, Dr. Blanchard increased the testosterone part of the cream, and I was so sexually hungry, it was like, come on! He lowered the testosterone. If I start feeling indifferent, I can let him know and he'll add some more, but he doesn't want to see me with a mustache and a beard!

If your "menopausal" symptoms are not controlled with estrogen replacement therapy (ERT), as was the case with Sherry, you may be among a large number of women over the age of forty who have an untreated underlying hypothyroidism. And when these hormonal fluctuations are brought back into balance, menopause can mean a change for the better, because hormonal replacement for menopause and hypothyroidism go hand in hand.

WHAT IS MENOPAUSE?

Menopause is a turning point in the lives of many women, representing many significant changes. It marks the end of the reproductive years and the beginning of a new era. If hypothyroidism complicates the picture, the change factor is doubled, and the hormonal rhythm that a woman followed for the past two decades loses its regular measure. Here's a look at what could be happening:

Physiologically speaking, menopause is your very last menstrual period. It's the time when your ovaries stop making enough estrogen and progesterone for a menstrual cycle. The ovaries usually stop ovulating a few years before cessation of cycles. Menopause doesn't usually hit all at once. It is announced by years, sometimes a decade or more, of fluctuating hormone levels. During this time, you might notice that you experience irregular periods, heavy periods, or scant periods that are closely spaced. However, this time of "perimenopause" also marks the time that your body starts to slow its production of estrogen.

It is the fluctuations in estrogen—not the reduction per se—that are at the root of symptoms. Acute (short-term) symptoms of bouncing estrogen levels include hot flashes and night sweats. These symptoms have a "cascade effect": The night sweats cause interrupted sleep, which can bring on fatigue, irritability, and mood swings.

The long-term risks associated with estrogen decline are osteoporosis and heart disease, as well as thinning of the vaginal and uterine lining and of the bladder wall. When the bladder wall thins, women may feel a greater urge to urinate or have difficulty in holding their urine. This is also a function of weaker muscles. Kegel isometric exercises can help prevent and correct this problem (see page 171), and testosterone skin cream is often remarkably effective in treating this problem. In addition, vaginal and bladder thinning can make you more vulnerable to bladder or vaginal infections.

Hormone replacement therapy (HRT), which combines synthetic estrogen and progestin, has been the mainstay of treatment for the symptoms of menopause. Today, based on the results of two landmark studies—the Women's Health Initiative and the HERS II trial—we know that HRT poses its own serious risks and should be undertaken with great caution in women considering long-term use. However, as we'll learn in the following pages, not all estrogens and progestins are the same, and when combined with thyroid hormone, they can be quite effective in helping women of menopausal age to feel a renewed sense of health and vitality.

MENOPAUSE AND HYPOTHYROIDISM

Based on symptoms alone, hypothyroidism and menopause can be difficult to tell apart: dry skin, depression, and weight gain. Indeed, hypothyroidism is most likely to emerge in women between the ages of thirty-five and sixty, the same years that frame perimenopause and menopause. And if left untreated, hypothyroidism can pose serious cardiovascular risks (see chapter 5). Coincidentally, this has been one of the clinical rationales for the long-term use of estrogen replacement—until recently (see below).

Part of the problem in distinguishing the two conditions is that they are closely linked. As catalysts for metabolism, thyroid hormones affect all cells, including the production of progesterone and estrogen in ovarian tissue. In addition, estrogens can reduce the effect of thyroid hormone and lock it out from receptor sites on tissue cells. As a result, thyroid hormone fails to reach its metabolic destination. In addition, estrogen increases the level of circulating carrier proteins, resulting in a shortage of free, active thyroid hormone.

It's Not All in Your Head: A Migraine Case Study

I've been hypothyroid since childhood. I felt fine for about twenty years just taking the standard T4 treatment. Then I was diagnosed with Graves' disease and received radioactive iodine, so I had no functioning thyroid. The doctors gave me T4, but I wondered: If the body makes both T4 and T3, why aren't they prescribing T3 too? Then, over the past ten years, I developed the most horrible migraines. I would take eight to ten Imitrex and *still* feel the migraine. By the age of fifty-four, I was still ovulating and menstruating. My uterus was a mess, but I couldn't seem to go into menopause. No one ever connected these symptoms to my thyroid condition. Or my migraines to menopausal symptoms. To every doctor, every endocrinologist, and every neurologist I'd repeat, like a mantra, "Don't you think that there's a connection between the fact that I have no functioning thyroid and I get these migraines?" They'd respond with their own mantra: "Your lab tests (TSH) are normal. T4 automatically makes T3. You don't need T3 or any other change in treatment." My son, who is also hypothyroid, found Dr. Blanchard's name on the Web. He immediately put me on the estradiol patch (0.05 mg), to be applied at the first sign of migraine symptoms. He also added T3 to my regimen. The most dramatic effect—and I'm sure if you map my brain you'd see it there—the most dramatic effect of T3 is that my migraines have lessened in intensity. I'm not stabilized; I've only seen him twice. But the effect was dramatic—as soon as he gave me T3. Now I can abort the migraine by taking the patch for a few days and one Imitrex.

I'll bet there are millions of women suffering from estrogen-related migraines who should think about thyroid as well. Unfortunately, most doctors scornfully dismiss it.

—Sylvia P., aged sixty-two

Sylvia's experience highlights the need for T3. Studies have shown that the neurological system is very responsive to T3 in its direct form—that is, T3 that has not been converted from T4 in the tissue itself. Sylvia's story also shows the complex interplay of hormones around the time of menopause. The inability to produce progesterone and stop her uterine bleeding was a direct result of her hypothyroidism; adequate thyroid hormone levels are needed to produce progesterone. Which is also why it's such an important factor in fertility.

THE ESTROGEN/PROGESTERONE CONTROVERSY: IS THERE A NATURAL ALTERNATIVE?

Clinicians and patients are at a crossroad regarding the treatment of menopausal symptoms. Two studies recently discredited the value of conventional HRT with Premarin (oral conjugated equine estrogens, 0.625 mg/day) and Provera (medroxyprogesterone acetate, 2.5 mg/day), the most widely prescribed combination therapy for menopause. Altogether, the investigators looked at 8,506 women on conventional treatment, compared with another 8,102 taking placebo. In brief, here are the results:

The HERS II trial investigated the effect of the estrogen and progestin HRT regimen in women with coronary heart disease (CHD) in preventing a CHD-related event, such as a stroke or myocardial infarction (heart attack). Not only did HRT fail to prevent CHD-related events, it increased the number of strokes and clots in the first year. The researchers concluded: "Postmenopausal hormone replacement therapy (HRT) should not be used to reduce the risk of CHD events in women who already have CHD."

In the Women's Health Initiative (WHI) trial, the same HRT regimen was studied to see whether it prevented CHD in apparently healthy women aged fifty to seventy-nine. After two and a half years, investigators began to see an increase in the rate of breast cancer among these women, and stopped the trial earlier than they'd originally intended. Investigators summarized their results by saying that conventional HRT "should not be initiated or continued for primary prevention of CHD."

Summary of HERS II and WHI Results

Measure	Percentage that Developed Problem Taking HRT	Percentage that Developed Problem Taking Placebo	Difference Between HRT and Placebo
Breast cancer	3.8	3.0	+26%
Clots	2.6	1.3	+100%
Colon cancer	1.0	1.6	−37%
Heart disease	3.7	3.0	+23%
Hip fracture	1.0	1.5	−33%
Stroke	2.9	2.1	+38%

REGAINING YOUR NATURAL BALANCE

As you can see, there are risks and benefits to using estrogen and progestin for menopausal symptoms. The long-term effects of estrogen loss must be addressed, as they can be debilitating or life-threatening: Bladder tissue becomes thinner, leading to bladder control problems; bone thinning is the cause of bone fracture; and heart disease is a greater risk for women as they age.

Recognizing these problems, I highly recommend natural hormone replacement. Even before the outcome of the above studies, I advocated and prescribed natural estradiol and progesterone, usually in lower doses than conventional HRT and delivered transdermally (through the skin via patch or cream) as an alternative to their synthetic counterparts. Unfortunately, the WHI and HERS II studies did not include natural hormones in their investigations, so we do not know how natural hormones compare to the synthetics. However, clinical data are quite positive, and separate studies of natural progesterone have found that it does not cause coronary artery spasm (as does medroxyprogesterone acetate); and it tends to lower high-density lipids (HDL cholesterol—the "good" cholesterol) much less than its synthetic substitute.

Natural Versus Synthetic Hormones

Natural hormones are biochemical, meaning that their chemical structure is identical to that of the hormones made by the body. Synthetic hormones, normally prescribed in conventional HRT, have a chemical structure that is foreign to the human body.

I can't say conclusively that natural estradiol carries fewer intrinsic cardiovascular and breast cancer risks—I don't think anyone knows for sure—but the dose I often recommend to patients gives a blood level about one-third of what is normally experienced during menstruation. And in the transdermal (cream) form, the route to target cells is more direct—it doesn't need to undergo metabolism in the liver or kidney.

In effect, based on the data I've reviewed, I believe that natural hormones are *less likely* to cause problems similar to those caused by synthetic hormones. Adding thyroid hormone helps further reduce the risk of cardiovascular complications. Ask your doctor about natural hormones. Finally, patients can take steps to guard their heart and bone health through diet, exercise, and nutrition. See below for some specific tips.

PHYTOESTROGENS: FRIEND OR FOE?

Phytoestrogens—foods that contain flavonoids, such as soy, uncooked cabbage, and flaxseeds—are highly acclaimed as healthful estrogen "substitutes." They seem to do everything from preventing the growth of breast cancer cells to improving many menopausal symptoms to lowering "bad" cholesterol. They're low in fat and high in protein. So they seem perfect not only for women in their menopausal years but also for women suffering from hypothyroidism.

There's only one downside: Phytoestrogens, like all estrogens, cause a decline in thyroid hormone levels. While I do not recommend that you completely avoid phytoestrogens, I do suggest moderation (as I do with nutrition and all nutritional supplements). I also highly suggest that your estrogen and thyroid hormone levels be tested *frequently* to achieve and maintain a healthy balance. This practice is supported in several clinical studies, including one recently published in the *New*

England Journal of Medicine, which recommends testing every twelve weeks. If your TSH results turn out normal—as is often the case, depending on the reference range for your local lab—pay closer attention to symptoms. Since T4 and T3 needs increase with estrogen use, you may experience more hypothyroid symptoms such as fatigue, bloating, headaches, and depression, requiring an adjustment in either estradiol or thyroid hormone dose.

OTHER WAYS TO ACHIEVE BALANCE

Balance requires temperance. By nature, extreme practices call for more effort to balance out. For example, phytoestrogens can help people with menopausal symptoms—and I recommend flaxseed to help joints and prevent heart disease—but in extremes they can reduce thyroid levels. I once had a patient who heard that fiber was good for GI symptoms of hypothyroidism and ate an entire bowl of bran each morning for breakfast. She lost a good part of her T3 and T4 dose that way—and all the benefits went down the drain, so to speak.

A balanced approach to managing menopausal symptoms that dovetails with your hypothyroid program includes the following:

- Do twenty minutes of daily exercise that leaves you slightly breathless (e.g., power walking, yoga sun salutations) to relieve night sweats and hot flashes.
- Take calcium supplements to slow the loss of bone mass in osteoporosis.
- Drink eight glasses of water daily.
- For vaginal dryness, try *water-based* vaginal lubricants or calendula cream.
- Avoid alcohol, coffee, and spicy foods.

- Consult with an herbalist about the right doses of black cohosh, red clover, hawthorn, and other herbs to cope with menopause/hypothyroid problems. See Resources, particularly Menopause-Metamorphosis.com, the Web site of women's herbalist Susun Weed.
- Try acupuncture, or speak with a doctor of traditional Chinese medicine about herbal remedies that may help to relieve the cause of menopausal symptoms.
- Take one or two 500-mg tablets of magnesium daily to reduce palpitations and migraines. Many magnesium preparations come with calcium.
- Do Kegel exercises daily to help restore blood flow to the vagina and bladder, strengthen these muscles, and improve bladder control. Here's how: Squeeze your vaginal muscles as though you're trying to stop the flow of urine.

SYMPTOM SIMILARITY: MENOPAUSE AND HYPOTHYROIDISM

As with hypothyroidism, not all women experience *all* symptoms of menopause. And as you can see, the lists of symptoms are closely intertwined. If your doctor is not convinced that hypothyroidism may be a significant factor in your symptomatology, show him or her this list. A family history of thyroid or autoimmune disease further substantiates your need for a diagnostic trial of T4 and T3.

Menopause Symptoms	Also Present in Hypothyroidism
Aching sore joints, muscles, and tendons	X
Anxiety, feeling ill at ease	X
Bouts of rapid heartbeat	X
Bloating	X
Breast tenderness	X
Changes in body odor	
Extreme fatigue	X
Depression	X
Disturbing memory lapses, difficulty in concentrating, disorientation, mental confusion	X
Dizziness, light-headedness, episodes of loss of balance	X
Dry skin	X
Gastrointestinal distress, indigestion, flatulence, gas pain, nausea	X
Gum problems, increased bleeding	
Hair loss	X
Headache change, increase or decrease	X
Hot flashes	
Incontinence, especially upon sneezing, laughing	
Increase in allergies	X
Insomnia	
Irritability	X
Loss of libido	X
Mood swings	X
Osteoporosis	
Skin disease, itchy, crawly skin	X
Tingling in the extremities	X
Urinary problems	
Vaginal dryness	
Weight gain	X

—•◆•—

Chapter 13

Keeping the Beat in Advanced Age

Emma, aged seventy, has been a patient of mine for over ten years. When we first met, she had been taking 2 grains of natural thyroid extract (Armour) for over twenty years with few problems. Her dose provided 76 mcg T4 and 18 mcg T3, in my mind a high proportion of T4—about 80 percent—to 20 percent T3. Six months before seeing me, she had gone to one of the eminent teaching hospitals in Boston and was switched to the "equivalent" of a "better" preparation, 100 mcg of Synthroid. Over the course of three months, she gained thirty pounds and experienced fatigue, brain fog, aches, and pains. After several visits, her new doctor agreed to put her on her old dose of natural thyroid extract. She felt no improvement and came to me. I was amazed that although her heart rate was high at 160 beats per minute, she was not in the least out of breath. Most people her age would be gasping for air. The reason behind Emma's success was the long-term effects of daily natural thyroid on her diastolic function.

Very simply stated, when the heart beats, the strength of

contraction of the heart muscle (systole) is followed by complete and rapid relaxation (diastole). With diastole, blood floods into the heart's chambers ready to be pumped back out through miles of arteries, vessels, and veins to oxygenate and feed every last one of the body's cells. The heart's ability to contract is reflected in the systolic function; its ability to relax is reflected in diastolic function.

If the filling part of the cycle (diastole) fails because of slow relaxation, then even a strong contraction can't pump enough blood to meet the body's needs. The ability to exercise, therefore, depends on the heart being able to increase the volume of blood pumped per minute. With a very healthy heart, exercise is made possible by increasing the heart rate. But when there's diastolic dysfunction, the heart rate rises with exercise while cardiac output drops, so not enough blood is reaching the body, and the ability to exercise is severely limited.

Many older people suffer from diastolic dysfunction. Emma's exercise capacity was excellent, in spite of her rapid heart rate. Natural thyroid extract had helped maintain very good diastolic function. Being somewhat T4-depleted on this dose allowed her to tolerate the high T3 dose without toxicity. But after three months on 100 percent T4, her tissue stores became flooded with T4, and the introduction of T3 caused clinical hyperthyroidism with rapid heartbeat.

I adjusted her doses to regain the balance she had achieved before taking 100 percent T4, now aiming for a physiologic dose with 2 percent T3 and 98 percent T4.

Emma has recovered her cardiac health and is a vitally active member of her community. Though I wish Emma had never gone through the weight gain and heart scare, she was relatively lucky in several ways. She had been diagnosed early enough to prevent severe cardiac problems, and her treatment included a proportion of T3, to which, although it was not a physiologic dose, she adapted very well.

HYPOTHYROIDISM AND ADVANCED AGE

As we age, our metabolic and immune systems begin to slow down, making us more prone to infection and immune diseases. Both effects can manifest as hypothyroidism. In older people, Hashimoto's thyroiditis is the most common form of hypothyroidism; in addition, many older people have subclinical hypothyroidism, which increases their risk of heart disease (see below). Studies show that by age fifty, 10 percent of women have signs of thyroid failure. By age sixty, 17 percent of women and 8 percent of men have a high TSH. Note that by age sixty, men are half as likely to be hypothyroid as women, whereas in youth, men are four to five times *less* likely to be hypothyroid.

The classic signs and symptoms of hypothyroidism in elderly patients are lethargy, fatigue, and dry skin, which are commonly associated with aging. In general, older individuals are also subject to the same symptoms as younger people, but they may be interpreted differently. For example, brain fog may be misread as dementia.

But one study showed that it's not unusual for older people to have a different set of symptoms. Up to 42 percent of men and women have atypical symptoms, which further clouds the diagnosis, such as behavioral changes, macrocytic anemia (large red blood cells), peripheral neuropathy (damage to the nerves, usually in the feet and lower legs), dementia-like behavior, and myopathy (muscle pain or weakness).

Cardiac Complications

Coupled with the risks of aging, untreated hypothyroidism can take a sizable toll on the aging heart. With cardiac awareness high among primary-care physicians, cardiac risks such as elevated "bad" lipids (LDL and triglycerides) and high blood pressure are likely to be picked up and treated in middle age—without investigating the underlying cause, hypothyroidism. Left untreated, hypothyroidism counterbalances many positive effects of treatment, and cardiac dangers stubbornly persist. So even though you might think that you've been keeping your blood pressure down or your cholesterol levels under control with medication, these conditions, if they're related to hypothyroidism, have probably been progressing nonetheless.

This pattern is most evident in subclinical hypothyroidism, where outward symptoms may not warn of underlying hypothyroidism. Older individuals with this form of hypothyroidism have a higher risk of myocardial infarction (heart attack) and arteriosclerosis (clogged arteries), according to investigators of a large study of more than fourteen hundred older men and women (average age: sixty-nine). Having thyroid autoantibodies alone didn't increase the risk of these life-threatening problems, but autoantibodies combined with subclinical disease raised risks slightly.

Atrial fibrillation is a common rhythm disorder in older individuals. The upper chambers of the heart (atria) contract at a very fast and uncoordinated way, resembling a trembling bowl of jelly. Some of the electrical impulses that filter down become blocked, so that the lower chambers (ventricles) beat at a slower rate—completely out of rhythm with the atria.

This condition is mostly associated with hyperthyroidism, but I suspect a hypothyroid origin in many individuals. In a monumental study of 2,575 patients over the age of sixty with atrial fibrillation, 101 of them had low TSH. Of these, about half were taking thyroid hormone, and of these 50 patients, 44 were found not to have hyperthyroidism. This is just one of many studies in the cardiac literature noting that atrial fibrillation presents with a low TSH but without other clinical or laboratory evidence of hyperthyroidism.

My rationale for a hypothyroid cause relates to excessive T4–T3 conversion at the cardiac muscle cell. This results in T3 hyperthyroidism at the level of the cardiac muscle cell, even though the patient suffers from hypothyroidism in peripheral tissues. It is of interest that the most effective drug to prevent recurrent atrial fibrillation is amiodarone, which is known to block T3 receptor sites in cardiac muscle cells. This hypothesis remains untested in my practice, since I feel it is too risky to add thyroid replacement in patients with cardiac rhythm disturbances.

Myxedema Coma

Myxedema coma is an extreme, life-threatening form of hypothyroidism that happens almost exclusively in older individuals (after age sixty) and mostly in women who are untreated. The vast majority of cases occur in the winter in tandem with other illnesses, infections, or severe stress.

Myxedema coma could develop after the patient is hospitalized and undergoes surgery because both events place severe stresses on body systems. In this condition, the first signs are drowsiness and cold sensitivity; soon the individual becomes unconscious, requiring emergency care. Adequate replacement of thyroid hormone is the only way to prevent myxedema coma.

Diagnosis Is Challenging

Joseph Knight, M.D., professor of pathology and head of the Division of Education, Department of Pathology, at the University of Utah, and author of the book *Laboratory Medicine and the Aging Process* (ASCP Press), identified four major problems in interpreting laboratory results:

- Subclinical hypothyroidism (early stage without symptoms)
- Other (nonthyroidal) diseases
- Multiple drug therapy
- Poor nutrition

These conditions can alter the results of tests to either mask existing thyroid disease or cause variations that mimic abnormal results in T4, T3, and TSH levels. When these complicating factors are excluded, the test ranges for younger adults can also be used for older individuals.

FINDING A HEALTHY BALANCE

My goal with hypothyroidism is the same for patients of all ages, including those in the older range: to eliminate symptoms through physiologic doses of T4 and T3. After a full evaluation for factors that might interfere or accelerate thyroid production (see above), I usually start patients with a very low dose (12.5 to 25 mcg) of T4 for the Two-Week Diagnostic Trial, paying close attention to changes in heart rate and blood pressure. In general, the doses of thyroid hormone need to be reduced as people age.

Among patients with moderate increases in TSH, many will have symptomatic improvement with this conservative trial of thyroid hormone replacement therapy. The most dramatic improvement is in patients with more severe disease. My patients and I are usually gratified to see layers of symptoms lift as thyroid hormones begin to take effect. What was once seen as the fatigue of old age is replaced by a newfound vigor. Dementia is replaced by a revived mental acuity and interest in the world. Movement becomes easier. Individuals reclaim their lives.

A Word on Pricing and Coverage

Although it is more expensive, make sure that your doctor prescribes brand-name thyroid hormone and that you fill the prescription exactly as written. Generics tend to vary in dose somewhat, depending on the manufacturer, possibly making it more difficult for you to reach the optimal dose and response, and requiring more office visits, more blood tests, more drug refills, more hassle, more expense!

You might save money by paying out of pocket for your thyroid medication. For example, some HMOs only dispense thirty days of medication at a time. It might cost you less to find a mail-order source and pay for the prescription yourself than to make a co-payment and pick up the prescription at the pharmacy (if you take a car service, for example).

PART III

The Care and
Feeding of the
Ailing Thyroid

I should begin this section by saying that I don't know of any truly effective alternatives to thyroid hormone for the treatment of hypothyroidism. When confirmed by a diagnostic trial, hypothyroidism fundamentally, and often critically, requires thyroid replacement. The focus of my approach derives from decades of experience with thousands of patients: the 2 percent solution—98 percent T4 with 2 percent T3, preferably with natural desiccated thyroid. A few patients respond beautifully to 100 percent synthetic T4; a few others do just fine with natural desiccated thyroid (which has a proportion of 80 percent T4 to 20 percent T3). Each person is unique and should be approached without prejudgment. A perfect example is my seventy-year-old patient Emma, who had the exercise capacity of a woman twenty years her junior.

With thyroid hormone levels in balance, I believe that most people could also benefit from a good daily multivitamin. Some may feel better with selenium supplements (see page 222). I endorse the use of flaxseed oil as a general nutritional supplement—I take it myself. I also believe that weight loss can be accomplished with a well-timed, well-balanced diet that is supported by a regular exercise regimen. My Thyroid Wellness Diet (chapter 16) reflects some of my basic beliefs about nutrition and metabolic rhythms. All of this is fine as long as you continue to maintain thyroid balance with hormone therapy.

That having been said, many of my patients are enthusiastic about "alternative" techniques that I haven't tried personally. They have my support to continue, as long as the method is safe. This means taking *recommended* doses of supplements or exercising *in moderation*. The concept that more is better applies no more to alternative therapies than it does to hormone replacement. Some may help you take the edge off symptoms, or lose weight faster, or help with your general well-being.

So in the following pages, in addition to my Thyroid Wellness Diet, you'll find personal nutritional supplements from patients. Homeopathic recommendations. Exercise regimens. General do's and don'ts. And more. I hope some of them work for you. A few guidelines:

- Keep track of your response and your progress. Generally, we rely on doctors to process this information from tests and symptoms—as I do with my own patients—and feed it back to us in the form of advice. But with alternative therapies, you will need to take the lead. It is up to you to keep in touch with your body's response and gauge your own progress, or lack thereof. A perfect example is the "Ten Hazards of Healthy Living" chapter, which shows how even the most scrupulous holistic health practices can backfire when it comes to hypothyroidism.

- Find a reliable partner in health. If you are working with an alternative therapist, make sure that he or she is truly qualified to guide you. See the Resources section at the back of the book for a list of organizations to help you find a skilled and competent individual.

Good luck and good health!

Chapter 14

Is Hypothyroidism in the Air?

When we think of the dangers of toxic chemicals, we usually focus on life-threatening illnesses such as cancer. But these serious diseases are an extreme end of the spectrum—the *most* serious consequence. En route, the accumulation of toxic chemicals can cause a wide scope of problems, ranging from bothersome to debilitating, including hypothyroidism.

There are currently more than seventy thousand chemicals in commercial use. Only a small fraction of them have been tested for thyroid activity. And fewer have been evaluated for their effects on embryos developing in the womb, which are most vulnerable for brain effects. In the words of Theo Coburn, author of an exhaustive review of environmental toxins, *Our Stolen Future,* "No human has been born since the middle of the 20th century without some exposure, in the womb, to hormonally-active synthetic compounds." I recommend the Web site OurStolenFuture.org as an updated source of information on thyroid-related toxins.

The chemicals of greatest concern are part of a group called endocrine disrupters. They have been shown in one way or another to disrupt the hormonal process. Some of the best-suited environmental endocrine disrupters are PCBs, insecticides, mercury, and fluoride. Others, which include a wide range of environmental pollutants, chemicals, and some metals, can be found on the Our Stolen Future Web site.

DDT AND THE XENOESTROGEN STORY

DDT is one of the most famous of a group of chemicals known as estrogen mimics or xenoestrogens—foreign ("xeno") chemicals that act like estrogens in the body. Bisphenol-A, a chemical used in the lining of food containers, and polyvinyl chloride (PVC), a ubiquitous plastic found in everything from test tubes to toys, are others. These fake estrogens include estrogens fed to agricultural animals that we in turn eat, plastic containers used for food and water, pesticides, and spermicides.

The relatively new area of study of xenoestrogens has uncovered an alarming number of disorders to which children are most vulnerable, though these disorders can leave a mark that continues into adulthood and old age.

What little we know about chemicals like DDT has alarming implications. Both animal experiments and human studies link behavioral disorders and learning disabilities with chemical exposure. When embryos and infants are exposed to certain environmental toxins during critical periods of brain development—that is, from one month in the womb to the age of two—the effect may be hypothyroidism-induced developmental deficiencies and possible permanent brain damage. And it doesn't take much to cause neurological problems. Very low-level contamination can alter thyroid function enough to impair brain development, according to one report. The undesirable effects can range from learning disabilities to attention deficit and hyperactivity.

As you may remember from chapter 2, most of the T4 and T3 produced by the thyroid are bound to proteins, which store them for later use. Because some environmental toxicants can compete with thyroid hormone for binding to these carrier proteins, the toxicants can lower the availability of hormone to tissue.

Based on lab tests revealing higher-than-normal thyroid autoantibodies, some investigators also believe that long-term exposure to certain xenoestrogens causes immune dysfunction.

KEEPING ENVIRONMENTAL HORMONE DISRUPTERS AT BAY

- Does your child's school pass the pest test? Parent involvement has often been the catalyst to reassess the need for using toxic chemicals in the school environment. Ask how pesticides are evaluated and which are used. Inform the school that you want to be notified when pesticides are applied.
- Eat low on the food chain. Select as many fruits and vegetables as possible in your diet. Animal fats, such as those in dairy products, processed foods, meat, fish, and chicken, tend to harbor toxic chemicals. Buy organic foods or simply lower fat intake by eating only low-fat animal products, such as nonfat milk and lean meats.
- Buy organic when possible. When not, peel and wash to remove surface contaminants.
- Keep your garden "green" by opting for the least toxic pest control method possible. This may include compan-

ion planting, mulching, and choosing pesticides with the least toxicity.

- Eat fish that is low in mercury. Unlike other chemicals, mercury inhabits the muscle of the fish, not the fat. High-mercury fish include swordfish, shark, and freshwater fish in contaminated regions (commonly found throughout the United States). Tuna, which is moderately high in mercury, should be limited to about six ounces a week (for a woman of average weight; see page 214). Before and during pregnancy and lactation, high- and moderately-high-mercury fish should be avoided in favor of fish like cod, which are lower in mercury.

- Clean up your household products. Use less toxic or nontoxic cleaning products. Avoid chemical dry cleaning, or at least air out dry-cleaned clothing before wearing it. Vacuum rugs often, which are reservoirs for pollutants.

- Eat soy and other phytoestrogen foods in moderation. See my Thyroid Wellness Diet in chapter 16.

Mercury

Hair loss, fatigue, depression, difficulty in concentrating, and headaches—are these symptoms of hypothyroidism, low-level mercury poisoning, or both? Studies show that mercury, a widespread pollutant, exists in high levels in fish—the same fish that people eat, such as salmon, swordfish, tuna, and shark. The Centers for Disease Control and Prevention estimates that about 8 percent of women of childbearing age have enough mercury in their bodies to pose a risk of having babies with mild learning problems. See chapter 16 for more on limiting mercury in the fish you eat.

PHYTOESTROGENS—THE ANTITHYROID?

Health food sages often extol the miraculous health benefits of soy: lowering the risk of osteoporosis, heart disease, cancer, and other maladies. While recognizing its potential, researchers are concerned about the hyperbole surrounding its role in a healthful diet. Experts especially question the safety of ingesting high doses of phytoestrogen, a mysterious ingredient that is now under local and national investigation. The claims swing wildly. One researcher espouses its value as a natural, nontoxic replacement for the now-condemned oral estrogen replacement regimen. Others, especially those concerned about thyroid health, see it as a threat to the thyroid—especially in infants on soy formula.

Not all of the soybean is bad, according to experts. Just the isoflavone portion—the part extolled by health gurus for its ability to prevent heart attack and reduce menopausal symptoms. Isoflavones are endocrine disrupters. Endocrine disrupters interfere with the endocrine system by acting like hormones and faking out the immune system. You might also hear about flavonoids, which is the family name for chemicals that include isoflavones (and bioflavonoids). On the flip side, these chemicals are known as goitrogens. Goitrogens fasten to iodine molecules in the gut—and steal iodine from T4 or T3. As a result, thyroid hormone levels are reduced.

The concerns about soy are widespread and fairly well publicized. The TV news show *20/20* picked up on the issue when two FDA soy experts, Daniel Doerge and Daniel Sheehan, wrote a letter in 1999 protesting the health claims for soy approved by the FDA. Here's an excerpt from the letter:

". . . there is abundant evidence that some of the isoflavones found in soy . . . demonstrate toxicity in estrogen sensitive tissues and in the thyroid. This is true for a number of species, including humans.

Additionally, isoflavones are inhibitors of the thyroid peroxidase which makes T3 and T4. Inhibition can be expected to generate thyroid abnormalities, including goiter and autoimmune thyroiditis. There exists a significant body of animal data that demonstrates goitrogenic and even carcinogenic effects of soy products. Moreover, there are significant reports of goitrogenic effects from soy consumption in human infants and adults.

The negative claims against soy are dramatic. One woman asserted that eating a high-tofu diet for just a few days a week set her menstrual periods off balance for three months. Faster brain aging, infertility, lower libido, and autoimmune problems (later in life among infants drinking soy formula) are just some of the reported problems, which many clinical authorities and, of course, the very profitable soy industry are disputing.

If you're hypothyroid, should you believe the bad hype about soy? The controversy rages and the jury is still out. In the meantime, it behooves you to limit your daily intake of this known goitrogen, as well as others.

SMOKING

If you've been hovering on the edge about whether to quit smoking, then maybe the following information will give you the impetus. Mary J. Shomon reports in About.com that smoking not only causes cancer, it induces hypothyroidism. We know that cigarettes contain much more than tobacco. And it is the presence of these additives that put the thyroid at risk. Cyanide (yes, the poison) in cigarettes converts to thiocyanate. This chemical assaults the thyroid by impeding iodide uptake. Other ingredients in cigarettes afflict the thyroid by interfering with T3 receptor binding and blocking its activity in organ tissue. The effects are cumulative: The longer you've smoked, the more severe the effects. There is some suggestion that long-term smoking may induce autoimmune activity. Long after the smoke has left your lungs, additives linger and accumulate, contributing to Hashimoto's and Graves' disease.

In a study reported in the *New England Journal of Medicine*, women with subclinical hypothyroidism who also smoked had higher total LDL levels than nonsmokers. Women with hypothyroidism who smoked also had higher serum cholesterol concentrations and more muscle problems than those who did not smoke. Researchers concluded that smoking impairs both the gland's ability to produce thyroid hormones and the hormones' ability to perform their metabolic duties.

FLUORIDE

Fluoride is added to over 62 percent of U.S. water supplies, according to the Fluoride Action Network. The aim is to reduce tooth decay, but mounting evidence indicates that, at best, it fails to protect teeth. A case in point: The water has been fluoridated in Newburgh, New York, since 1945. In nearby Kingston, New York, the water has never been fluoridated. Children in Newburgh have no fewer cavities than those in Kingston, but they do have higher levels of fluorosis—mottled teeth indicative of fluoride poisoning.

The toxic effects of fluoride on children are of gravest concern. One study compared the effects of iodine and fluorine on children's intelligence and metabolism. Children exposed to high levels of fluoride had a 17 percent higher rate of goiter than those in high-iodine areas (remember that iodine is a beneficial supplement for thyroid health). The dental fluorosis rate was almost double in the fluorine-exposed children (72.9 percent compared to 35.5 percent). Intelligence quotients were comparable between the two groups, but TSH levels were more pronounced in the fluoride group. But the most compelling evidence for avoiding fluoride if you're hypothyroid is that it has been used as a medication to reduce *hyper*thyroidism. Fluoride moves thyroid hormone levels in the wrong direction: *down!*

What can you do to protect your vulnerable hormonal system from the assaults of fluoride?

- If your water does not come from a well, learn about your community's fluoridation policies. Share information at public meetings to eliminate fluoridation.
- Drink unfluoridated bottled water. Read the label.
- Make sure that your water filter can remove fluoride— many do not.
- Do not allow dentists to apply fluoride coating to your child's teeth.
- Use a fluoride-free toothpaste, available at most health food stores.

Chapter 15

What You Should Know About Weight Gain and Hypothyroidism

Gina, aged thirty-six, seemed to be carrying the weight of the world. At more than 160 pounds, she looked heavy and dragged down. She also had been struggling for years with the emotional challenges of infertility and a hectic lifestyle. "I'd started to gain weight, but I attributed it to my insane schedule as a vice president and partner in a consulting firm. I traveled constantly and had to pull a lot of all-nighters."

Hypothyroidism was diagnosed through the fertility workup. Her doctor's solution to her problem, a dose of 100 percent synthetic thyroid, only seemed to help for a short time—and then things snowballed. "Headaches would wake me up in the middle of the night, I was exhausted, gaining more and more weight, and my hair started falling out—something was wrong. My doctor kept increasing the T4 dose because I couldn't seem to get enough."

Gina switched to a fertility/thyroid specialist who added synthetic T3 (Cytomel). "I didn't respond well at all!" she remembers. "I'd wake up in the middle of the night with palpitations and sweating profusely, so they stopped the Cytomel and upped my Synthroid dose to 175 mcg."

At this point, Gina delved into research and found Mary J. Shomon's Web site, which referred her to me. My first goal was to balance Gina's thyroid hormone by lowering her T4 dose and balancing T4 with physiologic proportions of T3. This would give her the foundation for starting a much-needed exercise program. I switched her from Synthroid to dye-free Levothroid to minimize allergies.

Over the next year, Gina started feeling better and better but had not lost much weight. By the end of a year, she was taking Levothroid along with thyroid extract in physiologic proportions. She felt much better and began watching her weight and exercising intensely.

The summer of 2002 was one of dramatic change for Gina. With her thyroid levels physiologically balanced, an intense kick-boxing regimen, and a low-carbohydrate, high-protein diet, Gina dropped fifteen pounds in three months. The impressive weight loss left her looking better, but not feeling as well as she could. I adjusted her dose slightly, reducing the T3 and increasing T4, and "it made all of the difference," Gina says. Today her TSH hovers between 0 and 1.0, her weight is 129 pounds, and she wears a size 4—down from a 12.

There are take-away messages from Gina's experience that are telling about thyroid disease and the challenge of weight loss.

BREAK THE VICIOUS T4 CYCLE: WEIGHT GAIN, HUNGRY FOR T4.

As I've pointed out before, T4 in toxic doses creates an unhealthy hormonal situation in people carrying excess weight.

At first, people taking T4 feel great as they experience a new infusion of metabolic energy. But over time, patients complain of fatigue and weight again and the need for more thyroid. This happened to Gina. Why?

Weight gain is a coping mechanism as T4 levels exceed the physiologic need, and TSH is suppressed. This reduces the conversion of T4 to T3. There's some evidence that fat tissues sequester the excess thyroid hormone to protect the body against hyperthyroidism.

A corollary to this theory is that the heavier you are, the more fat cells you have. This means, in essence, more cells to metabolize—the fat cells preoccupy T4 hormone. The other cells, in muscles, brain, digestive tract, skin, and hair, become deprived of the fat-consumed T4. As a result, you feel cold, tired, and mentally foggy; your hair falls out, your muscles ache, and so forth.

Many patients in this situation feel they need more T4, and as seen in Gina's case, many doctors believe the same. In fact, what they need is the physiologic balance of 98 percent T4 and 2 percent T3. I should note, however, that extreme obesity is a very difficult problem, and I do not have confidence that my thyroid regimen offers any real advantage over 100 percent T4. This is not the case with Gina, whose weight gain was moderate, and, though it took time for her to see results, the time was well spent in establishing a solid metabolic foundation that has allowed her to exercise and keep the weight off.

SLEEP YOUR WAY TO WEIGHT LOSS?

Gina's sleep-deprived lifestyle was not only making her tired and draining her thyroid hormone reserves but probably contributing to her weight gain as well. Physiologically speaking, in the early hours of sleep there's a significant rise in growth hormone, which helps break down fat and build muscle. By missing sleep—or even eating a high-carbohydrate snack before sleep—you're suppressing this metabolic charge. The blunting of growth hormone is worse in hypothyroidism.

In addition, as we saw in chapter 5, a recent study published in the *Journal of the American Medical Association* and the *Lancet* shows that sleep loss alters levels of cortisol, a hormone that regulates appetite (among many other things). As a result, sleep loss can make people feel hungry even if they've eaten enough. Moreover, sleep loss may interfere with the body's ability to metabolize carbohydrates and cause high blood levels of glucose, a basic sugar. Excess glucose promotes the overproduction of insulin, which can promote the storage of body fat, and can also lead to insulin resistance, a critical feature of adult-onset diabetes.

EXERCISE IS KEY

Exercise is key, but patient after patient has claimed that exercise is virtually useless in the face of a sluggish metabolism. For all of my patients who have lost weight, exercise was the complement to thyroid hormone balance. According to Gina, my program was "a real health saver. Every three months I return, and Dr. Blanchard tweaks my dosage based on how I'm feeling—for me, headache is a warning sign that I need a change."

Whether it's running, yoga, spinning, or kick boxing, a good cardiovascular workout has a cascade of positive effects:

- Improves metabolism
- Helps ensure better sleep
- Relaces fat with muscle
- Improves energy

The Rebound Effect and How to Avoid It

Weight rebounding is not a type of exercise program, but a term used to describe a pattern of losing weight then gaining it all back again. Rebounding is a common effect in organized weight-loss programs.

When weight is lost quickly, T4 hormone is ousted from its cushy home in fat cells. The result is a T4 rush—a virtual intravenous infusion of T4. The excess in T4 is sensed by the hypothalamus and the pituitary. The pituitary sends a message (via TSH) to the thyroid to put the brakes on T4 secretion in an attempt to protect against hyperthyroidism. T3 levels are also reduced, and the body achieves a certain equilibrium. But if you are taking 100 percent T4, the continual influx of thyroid hormone never gets balanced out.

In long-term programs to lose over fifty pounds, weight and thyroid levels need to be monitored closely with adjustments in T4 dosage, to avoid the hyperthyroid condition.

As the rebound effect occurs, the TSH is suppressed because of the previous weight loss—sometimes too low to measure because of the excess T4 released during weight loss. The physician is puzzled. Clinically, the patient is hypothyroid. But, in fact, the TSH is suppressed because of suppression during months of weight loss. Without TSH to stimulate the thyroid, levels of T4 slide back to hypothyroid levels, which encourages weight gain. TSH suppression under these circumstances also contributes to very low T3 production by the thyroid gland.

In my experience, the answer is to reduce the dose during active weight loss to keep the TSH level well within

> *the normal range.* This helps to keep T3 production going in the thyroid gland. When the goal weight is achieved, the T4 dose needs to be increased to somewhat below the original dose to avoid hypothyroidism, excessive hunger, and weight gain.

Thyroid hormone replacement is not a panacea for weight gain—it is a starting point. As you'll see in the next chapter where I outline my diet and nutrition plan in detail, rule number one is to balance thyroid hormone levels. Once you've achieved hormonal equilibrium, you're ready to venture out on solid footing to lose the weight you want—and need—to lose.

Chapter 16

Dr. Blanchard's Thyroid Wellness Diet

START BY LEVELING THE PLAYING GROUND

Metabolically speaking, people with hypothyroidism are at an innate disadvantage when it comes to weight loss. The first step is to balance thyroid hormone levels. Every successful hypothyroid diet plan hinges on this first step. By lifting you out of the fog of fatigue and inertia—and giving your muscles the energy they've been starving for—physiologic doses of thyroid hormone provide the metabolic push you need for a successful weight-loss program of diet and exercise.

EAT IN SYNC WITH YOUR NATURAL METABOLIC RHYTHMS

The worst thing you can do is to starve all day and save a thousand calories to ingest at night. When you don't eat, the body hunkers down and slows the metabolism to protect its fat stores—exactly the opposite of what you want to do! This common eating pattern works against your body's natural weight-loss rhythms, which are dictated by the release of growth hormone.

Eat Dinner Like a Pauper

While you're dreaming (or should be), your body is busy converting fat into muscle, thanks to human growth hormone. Human growth hormone is most active at night, especially during the first few hours of sleep. Do not disturb! The last thing you want to do is interrupt this natural weight-loss process by staying up too late or eating a lot before bed. If you must eat before sleep, opt for a small protein snack such as a skinless chicken leg. Protein takes longer to convert to energy, so it will fill you up and stand by without interfering with the metabolic processes at hand.

Eat Breakfast Like a King, Lunch Like a Prince

During the day, human growth hormone is not working as hard on fat-to-muscle conversion. This is the time to feed the body, so *start with a meal fit for a king*—a big, hefty breakfast is just what the doctor orders. You'll need the energy and you'll have the entire day to work it off.

Your medium-sized lunch should consist of a few hearty courses suitable for a prince. Allow yourself an afternoon snack—but keep it low in calories, low in carbohydrates and fat, and high in lean protein.

Select Thyroid-Friendly Foods

When preparing your food, try to minimize your use of thyroid foes, and select thyroid-friendly foods. Let your doctor know how much soy you eat so your thyroid replacement dosage can be adjusted, if necessary. Eating soy foods at the same time that you take your thyroid medicine may interfere with its absorption.

THYROID-FRIENDLY FOODS

Consume More Often	Consume in Moderation
Low-fat proteins	**Soy products**
Beef, lean	Edamame beans
Cheese, dry (low-fat string cheese, feta, goat cheese)	Soybeans
	Soy ice cream
Chicken breast	Soy milk
Eggs (preferably whites)	Soy protein powders and supplements (check for soy content)*
Fish: bass, bluefish, grouper, halibut, perch, salmon, scallops, shrimp, snapper, swordfish, tuna (canned; limit consumption— see page 214), whitefish	Tempeh
	Tofu
Pork	
Rice and beans	
Turkey breast	
Vegetables (low to moderate glycemic)	**Cruciferous vegetables**
Asparagus	Broccoli
Celery	Brussels sprouts (raw)
Cucumber	Cabbage
Green beans	Cauliflower
Lettuce	Kale
Onions	
Peppers	
Spinach	
Swiss chard	
Tomatoes	
Zucchini	

THYROID-FRIENDLY FOODS (continued)

Consume More Often	Consume in Moderation
Beans	**Root and starchy vegetables**
Black beans	Carrots
Cannelloni (white) beans	Corn
Garbanzo beans	Potatoes
Navy (red) beans	Sweet potatoes
	Winter squash
Beverages	**Beverages**
Water, water, water . . . as much as you can	Caffeinated drinks
Decaffeinated and herbal teas	Decaf drinks
Coconut milk	Sodas (diet and not)
Fats	**Fats**
Flaxseed oil	Butter
Olive oil	Lard
Safflower oil	Vegetable shortening
Nuts	**Nuts**
Almonds	Peanuts
Walnuts	Pine nuts

*One study reports of a woman who took her levothyroxine (T4) dose with a soy-based protein drink. The soy blocked absorption of levothyroxine, and the patient needed higher oral doses to maintain therapeutic TSH levels.

Eat a Variety of Foods in Small Quantities

Try not to eat the same thing too many times a week. Feeling restricted on a diet is a surefire way to break it. Shop with a general plan for your meals so that you always have healthful food in the house. An empty refrigerator combined with an empty stomach equals a quick carbohydrate fix. Try to keep potato chips, cookies, and other easy-access snacks out of the house entirely so that if you must, you'll opt for a hard-boiled egg instead of a bowl of corn chips.

MY THYROID WELLNESS DIET MENU PLAN

Consider the menu plan over the next few pages as a guideline—a way for you to sense how it feels to eat lots of protein, a little carbohydrate, and a lot less fat. Feel free to substitute your own favorites, or adapt with your preferred spices. Full recipes follow for the dishes marked with asterisks.

	Breakfast *Kingly portions*	**Lunch** *Princely portions*	**Dinner** *Pauper portions*
Sunday	Fresh or frozen blueberries ½ cup oatmeal 2 microwave scrambled egg whites 1 cup low-fat milk	Minestrone with low-fat Parmesan 1 slice whole-wheat bread	Salmon with Walnut Pesto* Spinach salad with feta tossed with Basic Vinaigrette*
Monday	2-egg red pepper and potato omelet 1 slice whole-wheat toast ½ melon	Tuna, Garbanzo, and Green Bean Salad* 1 slice whole-wheat bread Orange and apple salad	Lemon Broiled Chicken with Yogurt Marinade* Steamed asparagus with 1 teaspoon goat cheese
Tuesday	Cooked brown rice with almonds, walnuts, dried fruit, and low-fat plain yogurt 1 cup low-fat milk	Marinated Portobello Mushroom and Red Pepper Salad* ½ cup whole-grain couscous	Seared tuna steak Mixed grilled vegetables of choice tossed with 1 tablespoon olive oil, 1 teaspoon thyme, and ½ teaspoon salt
Wednesday	Whole-grain pancakes with fresh fruit Berry Smoothie*	Sliced turkey breast Tomato salad with parsley and cucumber tossed with Basic Vinaigrette* (omit the mustard) ½ melon	Vegetable lasagna made with low-fat cheeses and whole-wheat lasagna noodles Green salad

Thursday	½ melon
	¼ cup low-fat
	  cottage cheese
	Pineapple and Coconut
	  Tropicale*
		2 chicken breast
		  slices on low-fat
		  bread with mango
		  or tomato
			Grilled sirloin (4-ounce
			  serving)
			Roasted mushrooms
			  with sage
			Green salad

Friday	Whitefish spread
	½ toasted low-fat bagel
	Fresh berries
	¼ cup low-fat plain
	  yogurt
		Dr. Blanchard's Spicy
		  Bean Burritos*
		Papaya slices (when
		  in season)
			Fish of choice broiled
			  on fennel stalks
			Steamed green beans
			  tossed with oven-
			  toasted almond slices
			  and a dash of salt

Saturday	Eggs Florentine*
	½ grapefruit
		4-ounce low-fat
		  hamburger
		1 slice whole-wheat
		  or rye bread
		Tomato and green
		  onion salad
			Baked turkey breast
			  with cranberry sauce
			Roasted baby potatoes,
			  zucchini, and yellow
			  squash tossed with
			  1–2 teaspoons olive
			  oil and a pinch of salt

Healthful Snacks

Select from these protein snacks in midmorning and after dinner:

- Apple slices with low-fat cottage cheese
- Low-fat, low-sodium turkey slices
- Toasted almonds
- Vegetables with Creamy Sun-Dried Tomato Dip*
- Protein bar
- Low-fat cheese sticks
- Roasted skinless chicken leg

SELECTED RECIPES

Breakfast

BERRY SMOOTHIE

Serves 2.

1 cup low-fat plain yogurt
1 cup skim milk
1 cup fresh or frozen blueberries, strawberries, or raspberries
1 tablespoon honey

Combine all ingredients in a blender and blend until smooth.

PINEAPPLE AND COCONUT TROPICALE

This will serve 2 as a midday snack.

1 cup low-fat plain yogurt
1 cup crushed pineapple
1 cup coconut milk
1 tablespoon honey

Combine all ingredients in blender and blend until smooth.

EGGS FLORENTINE

Serves 6.

1 pound spinach, stems removed
1 teaspoon balsamic vinegar
1 egg yolk
2 teaspoons lemon juice
3 tablespoons butter

½ teaspoon salt (or to taste)
1 teaspoon fresh dill (½ teaspoon dried)
1 teaspoon white vinegar
6 eggs
3 English muffins, split
6 slices tomato

1. Wash spinach and boil for 3 minutes. Drain and squeeze out excess water. Set aside.
2. Heat a small frying pan over medium heat and add balsamic vinegar. Drop in egg yolk and stir. Add lemon juice, butter, salt, and dill. Whisk until creamy.
3. In a pot heat water over medium heat and add white vinegar. When water almost comes to a boil, add eggs and poach for 3 minutes. Remove with a slotted spoon.
4. Toast muffins and arrange on a plate. Cover each muffin half in this order: slice of tomato, spoonful of spinach, egg, sauce.

Lunch

BASIC VINAIGRETTE/MARINADE

Prepare and store this dressing as a marinade for roasted vegetables and chicken, or as a dressing for salads and grains.

Makes ½ cup.

¼ cup olive oil
3 tablespoons balsamic or other mild vinegar
2 tablespoons Dijon mustard
1 tablespoon lemon juice
Scant salt to taste
2 cloves garlic, crushed

Combine all ingredients and whisk until mixture thickens slightly.

MARINATED PORTOBELLO MUSHROOM AND RED PEPPER SALAD

Serves 2.

2 large portobello mushrooms
1 large red bell pepper
⅛ cup Basic Vinaigrette/Marinade (see page 206)
1 onion, sliced thin and roasted
1 teaspoon goat cheese (optional)

1. Preheat oven to 400 degrees.
2. Wash mushrooms and bell pepper and place in large mixing bowl.
3. Pour mixture over vegetables and cover. Marinate at room temperature for several hours (up to 48 hours).
4. Place vegetables in shallow baking pan and bake for 15 minutes.
5. Serve over couscous or make sandwiches on whole-grain bread. Sprinkle with goat cheese if desired.

TUNA, GARBANZO, AND GREEN BEAN SALAD

Serves 4.

1 6-ounce can low-sodium tuna, drained
1 6–8-ounce can garbanzo beans (chickpeas), drained
½ cup green beans, cleaned and steamed
1 tomato, chopped
3 tablespoons Basic Vinaigrette/Marinade (see page 206)

Combine all ingredients in a medium-sized bowl, mix well, and serve chilled or at room temperature with low-fat whole-grain crackers or pitas.

Dinner

DR. BLANCHARD'S SPICY BEAN BURRITOS

Makes 4 burritos.

Beans

12 ounces dried black or red navy beans
2 cloves garlic, minced
2 teaspoons fresh parsley, minced
1 teaspoon cumin
½ teaspoon red pepper powder (optional)

Soak beans overnight and drain. Place in skillet and cover with water. Bring to a boil and reduce heat. Add garlic and parsley and simmer, covered, for 1½ hours. Check frequently, adding water to keep beans covered. When beans are tender, add spices and cook, uncovered, until water has evaporated and beans are done.

Salsa

2 cups diced tomatoes
3 tablespoons chopped cilantro
½ cup chopped onion
1 tablespoon olive oil
1 clove garlic, minced
1 teaspoon dried thyme
Salt and pepper to taste

Combine all ingredients in a medium-sized bowl and mix well. Marinate at room temperature for at least 2 hours.

Burritos

2 cups cooked brown rice
1 tablespoon low-fat sour cream per burrito
1 green onion, chopped

Drain salsa. Place burritos in frying pan over medium heat for no more than 1 minute per side, just to soften. Arrange rice, beans, and salsa on the open burritos. Fold and heat for 30 seconds longer to meld flavors. Top with a dollop of sour cream and sprinkle with green onion.

SALMON WITH WALNUT PESTO

Serves 2.

¼ cup toasted walnuts
3–4 cups fresh basil leaves, washed and torn, with stems removed
2 cloves garlic
¼ cup olive oil
3–4 tablespoons low-fat Parmesan cheese
Salt and pepper to taste
Red pepper flakes (optional)
¼ cup chicken broth
½ pound salmon filet

1. In a blender or food processor, chop walnuts, basil, and garlic in oil until finely chopped to a "mealy" consistency. Add Parmesan, salt and pepper, and red pepper if desired and pulse just once to blend. In a thin, steady stream, with blender on medium, add chicken broth until the sauce is emulsified but still with some texture. Refrigerate, covered, until ready to use.
2. Preheat over to 425 degrees.

3. Place salmon in a large baking dish skin side down. Coat well with pesto. Bake for no longer than 15 minutes, depending on the thickness of the fillet, until center is a rich pink but not red. Remove and let sit for 5 minutes— the salmon will continue cooking for a minute or two. Serve warm. Tastes delicious the next day.

LEMON BROILED CHICKEN WITH YOGURT MARINADE

Serves 4–6.

1 cup low-fat plain yogurt
⅓ cup fresh lemon juice
3 cloves garlic, crushed
½ teaspoon paprika
Salt and pepper to taste
8 skinless chicken thighs or breasts

Prepare the first two steps the night before serving or early in the morning for dinner.

1. Sprinkle yogurt with salt and place in cheesecloth to drain overnight in refrigerator.
2. In a baking dish, combine lemon juice, garlic, paprika, and salt and pepper. Add chicken pieces and coat with marinade. Cover and refrigerate for at least 2 hours or overnight.
3. Bring chicken to room temperature. Preheat broiler or prepare grill.
4. Brush chicken pieces with yogurt and grill or broil until tender, about 25–30 minutes.

Snack

CREAMY SUN-DRIED TOMATO DIP

2 cups low-fat creamy cottage cheese
1 green onion, chopped
¼ cup minced red or green bell pepper
2 tablespoons minced sun-dried tomatoes
2 tablespoons fresh basil (2 teaspoons dried)
Salt and pepper to taste

Combine all ingredients in a blender and blend until smooth.
Serve with vegetables.

Chapter 17

Ten Hazards of Healthy Living: Holistic Habits That Could Make You More Hypo

Now that you've learned that you're hypothyroid, and you're getting treated for it, you have the energy for a renewed health campaign. Now's the time to be scrupulously healthy! But little did you know that many habits that are healthy for the general population can work against you if you're hypothyroid.

1. Eating Soy as Your Primary Source of Protein

Soy may taste great as tofu or tempeh. You may love soy nuts and edamane beans. Who can resist a Tofutti Cutie now and again? Whatever form it comes in, soy is an excellent low-calorie form of protein, and, for most people, it's a heart-healthy addition to the diet. But if you have hypothyroidism, go light on the tofu. Soy is known as a phytoestrogen and a goitrogen. This means that soy is like estrogen, a hormone that can interfere with thyroid hormone formation and activity. When consumed in large quantities, soy can contribute to hypothyroidism. In moderation (one fist-sized serving a day), soy will probably do no harm as long as you are also taking thyroid hormone. However, because it interferes with thyroid hormone absorption, soy should be taken apart from your medication. Allow three hours between eating soy and taking your T4/T3 supplement, just to be safe.

2. Drinking Bottled Water Exclusively

In the United States, you have to go out of your way to *not* get salt in your food or public drinking water. Which is what many healthy people do because of reports that salt increases your risk of heart disease. But by doing so, you're depriving your thyroid of one of its most important nutrients: iodine. Iodine is one of the building blocks of thyroid hormone. The "4" in T4 means four iodine atoms; the "3" in T3 means three iodine atoms. In iodine-deficient countries, hypothyroidism is epidemic. Goiters are a common abnormality. So if you follow the healthful habit of drinking only purified water, make sure to add a bit of salt to your food—and make sure that the salt is iodized.

3. Avoiding Salt in Food

The same rationale as above.

4. Drinking Raw Vegetable Juices Every Morning

A fine practice, as long as those vegetables are *not* broccoli, brussels sprouts, cabbage, cauliflower, or kale. These vegetables are rich in natural goitrogens, chemicals that interfere with thyroid hormone synthesis.

5. Ingesting Fruit When It's Out of Season

Unless you're buying organic (in which case the food is probably not as available out of season), you're purchasing fruits sprayed with pesticides that are illegal to use in the United States, such as DDT. DDT and other xenoestrogens mimic real estrogens, which interfere with thyroid hormone activity and formation.

6. Practicing "Safer" Sex with Condoms That Include Spermicide

A great idea in general, but not with the spermicide nonoxynol-9, which breaks down into phytoestrogens.

7. Eating Lots of "Freshwater" Fish

Fish are an excellent low-fat source of protein, but they can also be a source of mercury, an estrogen disrupter. To be safer, follow the guidelines below.

Fish Facts

Canned Tuna

The amount of canned tuna that is safe to eat *each week* should be based on body weight. Albacore and chunk light varieties have less mercury than solid white or chunk white.

25 pounds: 1 tablespoon
50 pounds: 2 ounces
75 pounds: 3 ounces
100 pounds: 5 ounces
125 pounds: 6 ounces (1 can)
150 pounds: 8 ounces
175 pounds: 9 ounces
200 pounds: 10 ounces

Fish That Have High Levels of Mercury
swordfish

shark

tilefish

king mackerel

tuna (steak)

Fish That Have Low Levels of Mercury

salmon	pollock
flounder	clams
cod	shrimp
catfish	scallops
trout	lobster

8. Using a Body Moisturizer Daily

Most commercial moisturizers contain paraben, which is a xenoestrogen. Daily application over warm, wet skin enhances its absorption. Make sure your moisturizer is paraben-free.

9. Having Spring Water Delivered to Your House

The large plastic containers that store spring water are lined with bisphenol-A, a xenoestrogen.

10. Taking Calcium and Vitamins

A definite and resounding yes for women over the age of thirty-five. But because calcium and vitamins can interfere with absorption of your thyroid medication, let your doctor know so that he or she can adjust your dose. Or simply take these supplements in the evening, or at least two hours after taking your thyroid medicine.

Chapter 18

◆

Top Tips from
Dr. Blanchard's Patients
(Plus a Few More)

Who better than my patients to reveal the most effective ways for people with hypothyroidism to lose weight and exercise? The following advice was gleaned from patients who have experienced gratifying weight loss and other improvements through exercise and diet.

The key benefit of exercise is that it stimulates human growth hormone and balances insulin levels. I do recommend that every exercise, diet, and supplement program begin with a talk with your doctor, who can help evaluate their safety and effectiveness for you as an individual.

KICK BOXING

Inspired by her newfound energy with Dr. Blanchard's thyroid replacement therapy, Gina started an exercise program that brought her from a size 12 to a size 4 and helped her lose thirty unwanted pounds. It's called kick boxing, a high-intensity workout that takes you through a professional fighter's training routine—and burns more calories than any other aerobic activity. It worked for Gina; it could work for you.

Activity	Calories Burned per Hour (180-Pound Man)
Walking	395
Circuit weight training	420
Cycling at 9 mph	490
Aerobic dancing	505
Swimming	630
Running	665
Basketball	680
Kick boxing	800

YOGA

When Michelle, whom we met in chapter 1, was thirty-nine and at the end of her rope, a yoga class brought her back—and saved her thyroid. She was facing thyroidectomy (surgery to remove her thyroid) when she tried a yoga class, and "immediately I noticed the mental clarity improve," she says. "Then I started sleeping better." Michelle attributes a big part of her progress to specific yoga poses and the overall sequence of poses used in a system that she now teaches called Bikram Yoga (also known as "hot yoga" because the temperature is kept very high to encourage flexibility and oxygenation).

"The other part of the equation was Dr. Blanchard," she says. "I felt good with yoga and my old medication. With Ken, I feel fantastic."

About Bikram and Some Thyroid-Specific Yoga Poses

The Bikram system of yoga that Michelle teaches is deliberately aimed at people of varied capabilities, especially those with health issues. It can be performed even by people who are overweight. Bikram is known for two things: its strict adherence to a specific twenty-six-pose *(asana)* series and for keeping the room very hot, often ninety degrees. The series is designed to warm and stretch muscles, ligaments, and tendons in the order in which they should be stretched. The room is heated to help facilitate deeper stretching, promote stress relief and toxin release, and prevent injury.

Inverted postures, where the hips are above the head, are particularly good for thyroid disease, as they help bring blood and oxygen to the thyroid. Consult your doctor before attempting shoulder stands or other inversions; and do not do them during menstruation.

DIET

Lynn describes herself as "pretty much a lazy person." Her favorite thing to do is planting herself on a couch somewhere to read or knit. But when it comes to diet, Lynn is no slacker. "Skim milk, wheat pasta, whole-wheat bread," she says. "My girlfriends' kids don't want to come to my house!

"My mom went on a health food kick in the seventies, and we never had good snacks in the house, so I try consciously not to be that extreme. But I limit the amount of bad snacks each day, and when we have a meal, it's well balanced."

Her approach works. Lynn lost twenty-five pounds with a good diet, exercising three or four times a week, and, of course, Dr. Blanchard's thyroid regimen as a base.

Debby is lactose-intolerant but believes in protein. Turkey, chicken, fish. "The more fish, the better for me," she says. "I stay away from carbohydrates, and I eat lots of greens."

Debby believes that people with hypothyroidism have trouble metabolizing nongreen vegetables and certain fruits. She avoids soy, even though she's lactose-intolerant. After working out at the gym, which she does three or four times a week, she sometimes allows herself a little hard candy.

SAMe: FORMULA FOR FIBROMYALGIA?

Penelope, whom we met in chapter 5, described herself as being at a pain scale of 8.5 out of 10; she couldn't open jars; she could barely walk around the block. Today she's traveling and working eight to ten hours a day. She attributes her life, her rebirth, to Dr. Blanchard's deep commitment to understanding her condition and to helping her. And Penelope also feels some debt to alternative treatments that might have contributed, such as SAMe.

SAMe is short for *S*-adenosylmethionine, a substance that occurs naturally in the body. It's a combination of two essential amino acids and plays a role in as many as thirty-five to forty biochemical reactions throughout the body. Usually, the body can make all the SAMe it needs, but patients with depression and other conditions such as fibromyalgia have been found to have lower levels of the compound.

The jury is still out at the Food and Drug Administration about SAMe, but European clinical trials have found SAMe to be as effective as some pharmaceutical treatments for pain and inflammation—a problem seen in fibromyalgia.

OTHER ALTERNATIVE TREATMENTS OF NOTE

In addition to the approaches endorsed by my patients, here are some that other individuals with hypothyroidism have found useful. Consider discussing these with your physician.

Homeopathy

According to homeopathic theory, the symptoms of a disease are an outward expression of the body's natural self-healing mechanisms; they are signs that the body is responding to the stress of the diseases. Using drugs to suppress the symptoms only masks the real problem and suppresses the body's own healing powers. In contrast, using agents with effects that are similar to the symptoms of the disease, homeopathic remedies act as a catalyst for the body's natural abilities. For hypothyroidism, *Calcaria carbonica* is just such a remedy. It has been found to be effective in helping with hypothyroidism, particularly if you are troubled by weight gain and menstrual difficulties.

Hydrotherapy

Hydrotherapy is the use of water of varying temperatures and pressures to alleviate pain and relieve tension. For hypothyroidism, a pattern called contrast application is recommended once a day to help bring blood flow to the thyroid, which aids in removing wastes. It also helps to stimulate the thyroid to produce more hormones.

With contrast application, the therapist uses terry-cloth compresses to apply hot and cold water in a sequence of four minutes hot (110 degrees) and up to one minute ice water. This is repeated three to five times.

Traditional Chinese Medicine

Traditional Chinese medicine is an ancient approach to medicine still vitally used to this day. It employs many methods—acupuncture and herbal therapy among them—to open channels called meridians which mark the natural flow of the body's elemental life force, or *qi* (pronounced *chi* as in *chief*). The meridians are the body's *qi* routes. In health, *qi* flows freely, enabling the body's different parts to operate as a unified whole. When the body is not in good health, there may be jam-ups or vacuums along the meridians that block the flow of *qi*. Stimulating specific points through manual pressure or the application of fine, threadlike needles helps to activate the body's own resources to overcome the problems. There have been several reports of excellent results with acupuncture for hypothyroidism. If you want to know more about traditional Chinese medicine, see the Resources section at the back of this book.

Massage

Massage therapy is not indicated specifically for hypothyroidism. But it can help relieve symptoms while you are undergoing thyroid hormone replacement. It is important to get your doctor's okay before having a massage.

NUTRITIONAL SUPPLEMENTS

Vitamin B complex helps to improve cellular oxygenation, strengthens the body's immune system, improves digestion, increases red blood cell formation, and aids thyroid function.

Essential fatty acids help to repair body tissues, aid in healing, and restore proper fatty acid balance, needed for healthy functioning of the thyroid gland. Essential fatty acids are found in omega fatty acids from fish oil, flaxseed oil, and borage seed oil.

Selenium deficiency can contribute to hypothyroidism. Selenium deficiency may occur in people who consume vegetarian diets or who eat foods grown from selenium-poor soil. Rich sources of selenium are liver, kidney, seafood, wheat germ, whole grains, and sesame seeds. It is important, however, to take the right dose of selenium. Excessive selenium is associated with depression of T3 levels.

Recommended Daily Amount of Selenium

Age	RDA (mcg)
Birth to 6 months	10
6 months to 1 year	15
1–6 years	20
7–10 years	30
Males:	
11–14 years	40
15–18 years	50
19+ years	70
Females:	
11–14 years	45
15–18 years	50
19+ years	55
Pregnant	65
Lactating	75

Source: R. H. Garrison and E. Somer, *The Nutrition Desk Reference*, 2nd ed. (New Canaan, Conn.: Keats Publishing, 1990).

Chapter 19

Finding a Doctor
You Can Talk to—and
Doing It Effectively

The right doctor can change your life, making the difference between health and hypothyroidism. It's worth spending the time to find the right one. In general, I believe that you want an open-minded clinician, either a willing primary-care doctor or an endocrinologist. Someone who makes a diagnosis beyond the TSH test. Who believes that managing your thyroid is a combination of TSH *and* how you feel, with sensitivity to ups and downs of thyroid levels at different times of life. In short, you want a doctor who will treat you like an individual, and not a lab value!

This is a fairly tall order in today's managed-care environment. But it's not impossible. It takes concern and effort. When you insist on individualized care, you are doing your small part to change the fixed vision of doctors who treat to the test, using only one therapeutic option, T4.

If your doctor does not seem to fit the bill, investigate other options:

- Meet other hypothyroid patients: there are local chapters of national thyroid educational organizations. (See Resources at the back of this book.)
- Check out the Internet. I suggest About.com's "Top Docs" section, which includes patient testimonials about doctors in different geographic areas.
- If you can travel, follow your doctor. I have patients from all over the world. After the initial input session, the doctor of your choice should be able to adjust your doses based on laboratory test results and symptoms, both of which can be reported from afar.

THE DOCTOR INTERVIEW

When selecting your physician ask yourself:

- Is your doctor receptive to new ideas? Ask about his/her philosophy regarding natural thyroid extract, T3, and adjusting doses based on symptoms versus lab tests.
- Does your doctor communicate clearly? You should be able to get a direct answer to your questions in a way that you understand. This is part of being patient-oriented, not numbers-oriented. If you don't, there may be a communication problem that could interfere with your future therapy. However, if the doctor seems to have an open mind about diagnosis and treatment, and seems genuinely interested in working *with* you, then these communication problems can be worked on.
- What is your doctor's philosophy about a "normal TSH"?

- How often will you be in contact? Will he/she be seeing you (or at least be in contact by phone) at least every six to eight weeks for a TSH test, followed up with an adjustment to your dosage, until you feel better?
- How available is the doctor/skilled staff between appointments? Is the doctor or his/her nurses available to answer questions? To address symptom concerns?
- Do you feel there will be an active partnership between you and the doctor in finding a solution?

HOW BEST TO COMMUNICATE WITH YOUR DOCTOR

You have a right to good health care. But any relationship is a two-way street. The way you approach your doctor can make all the difference in the way he or she interacts with you.

- Have confidence in yourself, being neither aggressive nor passive—you know how you feel. No one else can speak for you on this account. Do not let anyone convince you that your symptoms are not real. They are real to you and need to be addressed, whether or not the problems are ultimately due to hypothyroidism.
- Use your office visit to your best advantage. Write down your questions *in order of importance* before each appointment. You might make a copy of the list for your doctor and fax it ahead so that he or she is prepared to help you address them. Similarly, if you want to discuss a new study or article, send it off in advance so that your doctor has a chance to prepare (and doesn't spend your office visit reviewing it instead of treating you).
- Keep a regular log or diary of health-related events. If you are seeing a new doctor, bring a list of your previous doc-

tors' names and their addresses and phone numbers. Ask for a copy of your files from other doctors.

- Stay informed. Learn about the medications you are taking so that you can be an active partner with your doctor, and stay abreast of new treatments.
- Trust your instincts. It is your health and your life. Persist in finding the care you deserve. Don't settle for less.

WHEN SEEKING "ALTERNATIVE" THERAPISTS

With a skilled and knowledgeable practitioner, you may find that alternative therapies can really help you cope with symptoms while your thyroid medication is being adjusted, or as an added health benefit. Choosing a complementary-care practitioner also requires a careful selection process.

- Speak with your primary health care provider or someone you believe to be knowledgeable about alternative medicines.
- Ask basic questions about alternative practitioners' credentials, practice, and cost of treatment.
- Make sure that they feel comfortable sharing information about you with your primary-care physician or endocrinologist.
- Check with your insurer to see if the therapy will be covered.

For a list of holistic medicine practitioners and further information, contact the National Center for Complementary and Alternative Medicine (NCCAM) at (888) 644-6226 or nccam.nih.gov. Or for specific types of treatment, see the Resources section on the following pages.

Resources

———— • ◆ • ————

Arem, R. *The Thyroid Solution: A Revolutionary Mind-Body Program.* New York: Ballantine Books, 1999.

Coburn, T., et al. *Our Stolen Future.* New York: Plume/Penguin, 1996.

Conrad, C. *A Woman's Guide to Natural Hormones.* New York: Perigee, 2000.

Garrison, R. H., and E. Somer. *The Nutrition Desk Reference.* 3rd ed. New York: McGraw-Hill, 1998.

Landrigan P., et al. *Raising Healthy Children in a Toxic World.* New York: Rodale Press, 2002.

Lee, J. L. *What Your Doctor May Not Tell You About Menopause: The Breakthrough Book on Natural Progesterone.* New York: Warner Books, 1996.

Lowe, J. C. *The Metabolic Treatment of Fibromyalgia.* Lafayette, Colo.: McDowell Publishing, 2000.

Rosenthal, M. S. *The Thyroid Source Book: Everything You Need to Know.* 2nd ed. Los Angeles: Lowell House, 1996.

St. Amand, R. P., and C. C. Marek. *What Your Doctor May Not Tell You About Fibromyalgia: The Revolutionary Treatment That Can Reverse the Disease.* New York: Warner Books, 1999.

Shames, R. L., and K. L. Shames. *Thyroid Power: 10 Steps to Total Health.* New York: Harper Collins, 2002.

Shomon, M. J. *Living Well with Hypothyroidism: What Your Doctor Doesn't Tell You . . . That You Need to Know.* New York: Avon, 2000.

Wood, L., M.D.; D. S. Cooper, M.D.; and E. C. Ridgway, M.D. *Your Thyroid: A Home Reference.* 3rd ed. New York: Ballantine Books, 1995.

GENERAL INFORMATION

About.com
Thyroid.about.com
Comprehensive, patient-based resource.

American Academy of Clinical Endocrinologists
1000 Riverside Ave., Suite 205
Jacksonville, FL 32204
(904) 353-7878
www.aace.com
Resource for finding an endocrinologist; reviews of the latest clinical studies; medical search engine.

American Foundation of Thyroid Patients
18534 N. Lyford
Katy, TX 77449
(281) 855-6608
www.thyroidfoundation.org
General information for patients.

The Endocrine Society
4350 East West Highway, Suite 500
Bethesda, MD 20814
(301) 941-0200
www.endocrinesociety.org
Treatment and prevention of hormonal diseases.

Hormone Foundation
4350 East-West Highway, Suite 500
Bethesda, MD 20814
(800) HORMONE

Fax: (301) 941-0259
www.hormone.org
Information and resources about hormonal issues, including descriptions of different conditions.

Thyroid Foundation of America, Inc.
Ruth Sleepeer Hall 350
Parkman St.
Boston, MA 02114
(800) 832-8321
www.thyroidfoundation.org

Thyroid Foundation of Canada
P.O.Box/C.P. 1919 Stn. Main
Kingston, Ontario K7L 5J7
(613) 544-8364
Fax: (613) 544-9731
www.thyroid.ca

Thyroid Society for Education and Research
7515 S. Main St., Suite 545
Houston, TX 77030
(800) 849-7643
www.the-thyroid-society.org

ACUPUNCTURE

American Association of Medical Acupuncture
4929 Wilshire Blvd., Suite 428
Los Angeles, CA 90010
(323) 937-5514
www.medicalacupuncture.org

ALTERNATIVE THERAPIES

National Center for Complementary and Alternative Medicine
NCCAM Clearinghouse

P.O. Box 7923
Gaithersburg, MD 20898
(888) 644-6226
nccam.nih.gov

AUTOIMMUNE DISEASE

American Autoimmune Related Diseases Association, Inc.
Michigan Nation Bank Bldg.
14475 Gratiot Ave.
Detroit, MI 48205
(313) 331-8600
www.aarda.org

CHILDHOOD AND ADOLESCENCE

Congenital Hypothyroidism and Parents' Support Group
8 Rockhill Ct.
Edwardsville, IL 62025
(618) 692-1761

Magic Foundation (for children)
1327 N. Harlem Ave.
Oak Park, IL 60302
(800) 3MAGIC3
Fax: (708) 383-0899
www.magicfoundation.org

TRADITIONAL CHINESE MEDICINE

American Association of Oriental Medicine
(610) 266-1433
Fax: (610) 264-2768
www.aaom.org
See Web site for list of state organizations.

COMPOUNDING PHARMACISTS

International Academy of Compounding Pharmacists
P.O. Box 1365
Sugar Land, TX 77487
www.iacprx.org
See Web site to search for compounding pharmacists in your region.

ENVIRONMENTAL ISSUES

Center for Children's Health and the Environment
Mount Sinai School of Medicine, Box 1043
One Gustave Levy Place
New York, NY 10029
Fax: (212) 360-6965
www.childrensenvironment.org

OurStolenFuture.org

HAIR LOSS

American Hair Loss Council
125 7th St., Suite 625
Pittsburgh, PA 15222
(800) 274-8717
(412) 765-3666
Fax: (412) 765-3669
www.ahlc.org

INFERTILITY

Fertility Research Foundation, Inc.
877 Park Ave.
New York, NY 10021
(212) 744-5500

Resolve, Inc.
1310 Broadway
Somerville, MA 02144
(617) 623-9744
www.resolve.org

MENOPAUSE

Menopause-Metamorphosis.com
Susun Weed
P.O. Box 64
Woodstock, NY 12498
www.susunweed.com
Alternative approaches to menopause.

North American Menopause Society
P.O. Box 94527
Cleveland, OH 44101
(440) 442-7550
www.menopause.org

YOGA

Bikram Yoga
1862 S. La Cienega Blvd.
Los Angeles, CA 90035
(310) 854-5800
Fax: (310) 854-6200
www.bikramyoga.com

Yoga Research and Education Center
(and International Association of Yoga Therapists)
2400A County Center Dr.
Santa Rosa, CA 95403
(707) 566-9000
www.yrec.org

Glossary

———————— •◆• ————————

Ablate—to remove or to destroy the function of an organ or tissue. Radioactive iodine treatment ablates thyroid tissue.

Addison's disease—a disease of the adrenal glands, which causes a deficiency in the secretion of adrenocorticol hormones. Symptoms include low blood pressure, weight loss, anorexia, weakness, and increased pigmentation of the skin. It is treated with adrenal hormone replacement therapy.

Adrenal glands—two small glands that sit on top of each kidney. They release hydrocortisone, which affects metabolism. They also produce androgen hormones and aldosterone, which maintains blood pressure and the body's salt and potassium balance.

Alopecia—the absence or loss of hair due to serious illness, endocrine disorders, or radiation therapy.

Anemia—a reduction in the number of circulating red blood cells in the body. Red blood cells are important for transporting oxygen to the cells to create energy. It is a symptom of a disease, not a disease. Symptoms include pale skin, weakness, fatigue, and angina pectoris.

Anovulation—the absence of ovulation, or egg production, in a woman's reproductive cycle.

Antithyroid agents—drugs that block the production of thyroid hormones by the thyroid gland. Tapazole (methimazole) and propylthiouracil are examples of antithyroid drugs.

Antithyroid antibodies—antibodies that act against the tissues in the thyroid gland; also called antithyroid autoantibodies.

Asthenia—lack or loss of muscle strength.

Autoantibodies—*see* Antithyroid antibodies.

Autoimmune disease—a condition in which the body's immune system attacks its own tissues or organs.

Basal metabolic rate (BMR)—the rate of metabolism, or how fast the body uses calories and oxygen to produce energy. Hormones produced by the thyroid affect this rate.

Benign—the word used to describe a nonmalignant growth or mild illness.

Biopsy—a procedure where a small piece of tissue is removed from the patient for microscopic analysis to establish a precise diagnosis.

Bradycardia—a slow heartbeat characterized by a pulse rate of fewer than sixty beats per minute.

Calcitonin—a hormone produced by the thyroid gland which produces a strong bone matrix and regulates the level of calcium in the blood.

Carpal tunnel syndrome—a pain and/or numbness in the hands or wrists, usually due to the effect of cumulative trauma.

CAT scan—*see* CT scan.

Clearance—the normal elimination of a substance from the blood by the kidneys.

Cold nodule—a lump in the thyroid gland that is seen on a scan because it does not take up as much radioactive iodine as the surrounding tissue.

Computerized rectilinear thyroid (CRT) scanner—the preferred instrument used today for thyroid screening.

Congenital hypothyroidism—a rare condition among newborn infants in which improper growth of the thyroid gland results in insufficient amount of thyroid hormone. Serious developmental effects can occur, such as slow growth and reduced mental function, as well as cardiac abnormalities. These consequences usually, but not always, can be avoided or minimized with early diagnosis and treatment with thyroid hormone replacement.

Congestive heart failure—when the heart is not working properly, it is unable to pump all the blood it receives. This causes fluid in the blood to back up in the lungs, liver, abdomen, and legs. This backup of fluid is called congestive heart failure.

Constipation—a state in which one experiences a reduced change in the frequency of one's own bowel habits. Normal bowel habits differ widely between individuals (from two or three times a day to two or three times a week).

Controlled clinical trials—studies in which results observed in patients receiving a drug are compared to the results in patients who did not receive the drug.

Count—a unit of measurement used to gauge levels of radioactivity.

CT scan—computerized axial tomographic scan; an imaging procedure also called a CAT scan. It is useful for the evaluation and follow-up of thyroid cancer patients and assessing the extent of metastatic and vascular invasion. It is not useful in differentiating benign from malignant nodules.

Deiodinase—an enzyme that helps convert T4 to T3.

Desiccated pig extract—thyroid glands from pigs (who have already been slaughtered for other purposes) that have been processed for taking as a pill.

Developmental delay—a delay in reaching the milestones of early childhood development.

Diffuse goiter—an enlargement of the entire thyroid gland.

Endocrine disrupter—any chemical that disrupts the normal functioning of the endocrine system (glands and hormones), which regulates a wide range of biological processes.

Endocrine glands—glands that secrete hormones into the bloodstream, which can have a specific effect on a tissue or organ, or a generalized effect on the whole body.

Endocrinologist—physician who specializes in the care of patients with disorders of the endocrine glands.

Endocrinology—the study of diseases and disorders of the endocrine system (like thyroid diseases and diabetes). The endocrine system consists of glands that release hormones directly into the blood. The purpose of secreted hormones is to evoke a specific response in other faraway cells.

Estrogen—a hormone produced predominantly by the ovaries, responsible for the development of female secondary sex characteristics and preparing the uterus for childbearing.

Euthyroid—having a thyroid gland that functions normally.

Euthyroidism—the condition of having the proper amount of thyroid hormone in the body.

Excipient—an additive to a product to improve it in some way; excipients in certain doses of thyroid hormone replacement can cause allergies.

Fatigue—a feeling of weariness, sleepiness, or irritability following a period of physical or mental activity, which results in a reduced capacity for work or accomplishment.

Follicles—microscopic spherical units that make up the thyroid gland.

Follicular cancer—a type of cancer made up of thyroid follicular cells; also called follicular carcinoma. Follicular cancer is a type of well-differentiated thyroid cancer, which means that the malignant cells closely resemble thyroid tissue.

Free T4—the amount of T4 (thyroxine) in the bloodstream that is not bound to carrier proteins. T4 is a hormone produced by the thyroid gland.

Free thyroxine index (FT1 or T7)—a calculation using T4 resin uptake and T4 to estimate the amount of T4 in the bloodstream. This can help to determine how well the thyroid is functioning.

Galactorrhea—the continuing production of milk after nursing has ceased.

Gamma camera—an instrument that produces images of the thyroid glands after the oral administration of radioactive materials.

Glucose—a common monosaccharide that is a component of disaccharide (sucrose, lactose, and maltose) and various complex carbohydrates. It is also the end product of carbohydrate metabolism and the chief source of energy in the body. Its utilization is controlled by insulin (a hormone produced by the pancreas).

Goiter—an enlargement of the thyroid gland for any reason. It may be a generalized enlargement (diffuse) or asymmetric (nodular).

Goitrogen—a substance that causes enlargement of the thyroid, such as soy.

Graves' disease—a disease of unknown origin characterized by hyperthyroidism (with a diffuse goiter). Other symptoms may include eyes that appear to be popping out of their sockets and warm, moist skin with a velvety feel.

Hashimoto's autoimmune thyroiditis—a chronic inflammation of the thyroid caused by the immune system attacking its own tissues; also known as Hashimoto's disease. It often causes a goiter and results in hypothyroidism. Usually treated with thyroid replacement therapy.

HDL—high-density lipoprotein, a measure of cardiovascular health. An elevated HDL with a low LDL is indicative of healthy cholesterol balance.

Hoarseness—an unnaturally deep or rough quality of voice.

Hormones—chemicals produced by an endocrine gland and released into the blood. Hormones travel to other organs of the body, where they can produce their effect (increasing or decreasing functional activity). They can also be produced artificially and used to treat patients whose bodies are unable to produce hormones.

Hot nodule—a lump in the thyroid gland that takes up more radioactive iodine on a scan than the normal surrounding thyroid tissue. Hot nodules are rarely cancerous.

hTSH—human thyroid-stimulating hormone.

Hürthle cell cancer—a form of follicular thyroid cancer.

Hyperthyroidism—a condition in which the thyroid gland produces increased amounts of thyroid hormone. Symptoms are associated with an increased metabolism and include weight loss, increased blood pressure, and anxiety.

Hypo—a familiar term for hypothyroidism.

Hypothalamic-pituitary-thyroid axis—a negative feedback mechanism through which hormone secretion is regulated. The hypothalamus secretes a releasing hormone (TRH) that stimulates the pituitary to secrete thyroid-stimulating hormones, which then enter the circulation.

Hypothalamus—an endocrine gland in the brain that secretes thyrotropin-releasing hormone (TRH) and regulates autonomic activities such as body temperature and certain metabolic processes.

Hypothyroidism—a condition in which the thyroid gland produces insufficient quantities of thyroid hormone. Symptoms include obesity, dry skin and hair, an overall sluggishness of body functions, and a marked sensitivity to cold. It is treated with hormone replacement therapy and, if necessary, by increasing the intake of dietary iodine.

Impotence—an inability to achieve or sustain a penile erection.

Insulin—a hormone secreted by the pancreas in response to high blood sugar levels. It stimulates the uptake of blood glucose into cells, the formation of glycogen in the liver, and various other processes. Defective secretion of insulin is the cause of diabetes mellitus.

Iodine—a nonmetallic element found in food that is necessary for the production of thyroid hormone and for normal thyroid functioning.

Isthmus—a small piece of tissue that connects the right and left lobes of the thyroid.

Larnyx—the upper part of the trachea that contains the vocal cords, sometimes called the voice box.

LDL—low-density lipoprotein ("bad" cholesterol). The higher the LDL levels in the blood, the greater the risk for coronary heart disease.

Levothyroxine sodium—thyroid hormone supplement. Examples of brand-name levothyroxine pills are Synthroid, Levoxyl, Levothroid, and Unithroid.

Lobectomy—surgical removal of all of one lobe or part of one lobe of the thyroid. Indicated in some cases of thyroid cancer.

Lobes—the halves of the thyroid gland that give it its butterfly-like shape. The right lobe is often slightly larger than the left lobe.

Lymph nodes—small bean-shaped structures scattered along the vessels of the lymphatic system. The lymph nodes produce white blood cells and filter bacteria and cancer cells that may travel through the system.

Lyophilization—freeze-drying. The process of isolating a solid substance from solution by freezing the solution and evaporating the ice under vacuum.

Magnetic resonance imaging (MRI)—an imaging procedure that produces a clear three-dimensional picture.

Medullary thyroid cancer—thyroid cancer arising from the parafollicular cells. Although it grows slowly, it may be harder to control than papillary and follicular tumors. It is more aggressive than well-differentiated thyroid cancer and tends to spread to other parts of the body.

Menorrhagia—excessive and extended uterine bleeding during the menstrual cycle.

Metabolism—the use of calories and oxygen to produce energy in the body.

Metastatic disease—cancer that has spread from its original site to other parts of the body via the bloodstream or lymphatic system.

Mortality rate—death rate.

MRI—*see* Magnetic resonance imaging.

Multinodular goiter—a goiter in which the enlargement consists of multiple lumps.

Myasthenia gravis—a disease usually affecting the muscles of the eyes, face, lips, tongue, throat, or neck, causing muscle weakness, disability, and fatigue.

Myxedema—a condition caused by the thyroid gland producing grossly insufficient amounts of thyroid hormone (hypothyroidism).

Myxedema coma—a rare complication of severe hypothyroidism associated with hypoventilation (insufficient breathing), increased levels of carbon dioxide in the blood, low oxygenation, and low blood pressure. It is a life-threatening emergency.

Myxedema madness—psychosis associated with severe hypothyroidism.

Non-insulin-dependent diabetes mellitus—a mild form of diabetes mellitus of gradual onset after the age of thirty-five. Usually associated with obesity. It responds well to dietary changes.

Obesity—a marked increase in body weight beyond the limitation of skeletal and physical requirement, due to an excessive accumulation of fat in the body.

Obstructive sleep apnea—a sudden, temporary stopping of normal breathing while sleeping.

Ovaries—female glands that produce the reproductive cell (ovum) and two hormones, estrogen and progesterone, responsible for the development and maintenance of female secondary sex characteristics, preparing the uterus for pregnancy and the development of the mammary gland.

Pancreas—the abdominal organ that secretes insulin and glucagon and controls the utilization of sugar to create energy.

Papillary cancer—a well-differentiated thyroid cancer composed of thyroid follicular cells. Also called papillary carcinoma.

Parathyroid glands—four glands located on the back of the thyroid that produce parathyroid hormone, which controls the metabolism of calcium and phosphorus.

Paresthesia—burning, prickling, or tingling sensation in the skin.

Pericardial effusion—a collection of fluid inside the pericardial sac (which surrounds the heart) due to congestive heart failure, cancer, or autoimmune disorders.

Pernicious anemia—a deficiency of red blood cells essential for the transportation of oxygen to the cells of the body, due to an inability to absorb B_{12} from the gastrointestinal tract.

PET (positron emission tomography) scan—an imaging technique that uses radioactive positrons (positively charged particles) to detect subtle changes in the body's metabolism and chemical activities.

Petechiae—small red spots due to tiny hemorrhages within the skin.

Phytoestrogens—estrogen-like compounds that occur naturally in certain plants and fungi (soybeans, yams, citrus fruits) and are biologically active in humans and animals.

Pineal gland—a cone-shaped gland at the base of the brain that secretes the hormone melatonin, which may help to synchronize biorhythms and mark the passage of time.

Pituitary gland—a small gland the size of a peanut located behind the eyes at the base of the brain that signals other glands to secrete hormones. It secretes thyroid-stimulating hormone (TSH), which helps control thyroid function, as well as other hormones involved in endocrine function.

Placebo—an inactive substance that looks, smells, and tastes the same as a drug in a clinical study.

Pleural effusion—a collection of fluid/blood in the pleural space (around the lung) as a result of trauma, cancer, or other diseases.

Postpartum depression—depression that occurs after giving birth.

Postpartum thyroiditis—an inflammation of the thyroid occurring after giving birth.

Potassium iodide—a drug used to treat certain thyroid disorders. It can also be used to block the uptake by the thyroid of radioactive iodine isotopes that are released in a nuclear-reactor accident.

Progesterone—a hormone produced by the corpus luteum in the ovary that prepares the uterus for pregnancy.

Prognostic indicators—factors that can help predict a likely outcome (as in how, on average, thyroid cancer will progress).

Quality of life (QOL)—a person's physical, mental, and social well-being. Also known as health-related quality of life (HRQOL).

Radioactive iodine uptake (RAIU)—a test measuring the percentage of orally administered radioactive iodine taken up by the thyroid gland.

Radioactive isotopes—unstable chemical elements that are used in diagnostic testing for thyroid disorders, including thyroid cancer.

RAI ablation—the administration of a radioactive form of iodine (I-311) to try to destroy any remnant (normal or cancerous) thyroid tissues left after surgery in the thyroid bed or neck.

Receptor—a molecular structure within a cell or on the surface of a cell that selectively binds to specific substances.

Recombinant DNA technology—the technique of isolating genes from one organism and purifying and reproducing them in another organism. Sometimes called genetic engineering.

Rheumatoid arthritis—a chronic inflammatory disease of the joints (possibly an autoimmune disorder) characterized by stiffness, loss of mobility, weakness, and deformity.

Scintigraphy—a diagnostic procedure using a radioactive agent with affinity for the tissue of interest, followed by a whole body scan.

Secondary hypothyroidism—hypothyroidism that occurs as a consequence of inadequate amounts of thyrotropin secreted by the pituitary gland.

Secretion—the substance produced by a glandular organ.

Sensitivity—the ability of a test to detect the proportion of true positive results from the disease that the test is intended to reveal. In other words, the probability that, given the presence of disease, a test result will indicate that presence.

Signs—those characteristics that a physician can objectively detect or measure. If the physician touches the patient's skin and notes that it is warm and moist, this is a sign. *See also* Symptoms.

Specificity—the ability of a test to detect the proportion of true negative results for the disease that the test is intended to reveal. In other words, the probability that, given the absence of disease, a test result will exclude the disease.

Standardized—using different techniques or preparations in order to conform to a reference or standard.

Statistics—the study of probabilities. Statistics are used in clinical trials to determine whether results obtained with the study are truly different from those obtained with the control (or placebo).

Subclinical hypothyroidism—a mildly elevated TSH level with normal T3 and T4 levels.

Symptoms—those problems that a patient notices or feels. If a patient feels hot, this is a symptom. *See also* Signs.

Systemic lupus erythematosus—an autoimmune disease whereby the body's immune system attacks itself. Symptoms include joint pain, stiffness or swelling, fever, weight loss, fatigue, and a butterfly rash on the face.

T3 (triiodothyronine)—the metabolically active hormone produced by the thyroid gland by the breakdown of thyroxine (T4).

T4 (thyroxine)—the primary hormone produced by the thyroid gland. Naturally formed from iodine atoms, this hormone circulates through the body primarily bound to carrier proteins. It functions to regulate metabolism.

Testes—male reproductive glands that secrete testosterone, which stimulates sperm production and the development of male characteristics.

Tg test—a test that measures the level of thyroglobulin (Tg) in the blood. Tg tests are used in the postsurgical monitoring of thyroid cancer patients to check for thyroid remnants or cancer metastases.

Thrombocytopenic purpura—a rare autoimmune disorder in which blood platelets (important for clotting the blood) are reduced in number, which may lead to bleeding disorders.

Thyroglobulin (Tg)—a large protein that acts as a storage site for thyroid hormones within the thyroid gland. Following surgical removal of a cancerous thyroid gland, the level of Tg in the bloodstream can be monitored to detect thyroid cancer recurrence.

Thyroglobulin antibodies (TgAb)—autoantibodies produced by the body against its own thyroglobulin proteins. TgAb attacks the thyroid and disrupts thyroid function.

Thyroid—a two-lobed gland lying at the base of the throat that controls metabolism through the secretion of hormones (T4 and T3).

Thyroid bed—the area of the thyroid that remains after surgical removal of the thyroid gland.

Thyroid-binding proteins—proteins to which thyroid hormones attach themselves and thus circulate in the bloodstream.

Thyroid cancer—a rare thyroid disease characterized by uncontrolled tissue proliferation in the thyroid. Can occur in people who have been exposed to radiation.

Thyroid Hormone Binding Ratio (THBR)—recommended nomenclature for a T3 uptake test.

Thyroid hormones—T4 (triiodothyronine) and T3 (thyroxine), two hormones produced by the thyroid gland essential to regulating growth and rate of metabolism.

Thyroid hormone suppression therapy (THST)—in patients who have had a thyroidectomy for thyroid cancer, physicians usually prescribe a moderate excess of thyroid hormones to create a negative feedback loop that suppresses thyroid-stimulating hormone production by the pituitary gland. TSH production is suppressed to avoid stimulating existing thyroid remnants or thyroid cancer cells.

Thyroid nodules—masses (usually benign) that can form in the thyroid gland and may produce excessive thyroid hormone. In a normal gland or a multinodular goiter, thyroid nodules may be solitary or multiple. Imagine tests, blood tests, and fine-needle aspiration biopsies (FNAB) are used to perform a clinical evaluation of thyroid nodules.

Thyroid peroxidase (TPO)—a protein found in thyroid follicle cells that catalyze the iodination of T4 and T3 in thyroid hormone biosynthesis.

Thyroid peroxidase antibodies (TPOAb)—autoantibodies produced by the body against its own thyroid peroxidase enzymes. TPOAb attacks the thyroid and disrupts thyroid function.

Thyroid remnant—some part of the original thyroid gland remaining after thyroidectomy surgery.

Thyroid scan—a picture of the thyroid gland obtained with a rectilinear scanner and radioactive materials.

Thyroid stimulating hormone (TSH)—a pituitary hormone (thyrotropin) that promotes growth of the thyroid gland and stimulates the thyroid gland to secrete hormones.

Thyroid ultrasound—a type of scan that uses sound waves, which pass into the body and reflect back to produce images.

Thyroidectomy—surgical removal of the thyroid gland.

Thyroiditis—an inflammation (not an infection) of the thyroid gland. There are several forms of thyroiditis, including chronic. Hashimoto's thyroiditis, subacute thyroiditis, and painless or postpartum thyroiditis, and the treatment is different for each.

Thyroidologists—doctors who specialize in the treatment of diseases of the thyroid.

Thyrotropin—another name for thyroid-stimulating hormone (TSH).

Thyrotropin-releasing hormone (TRH)—a hormone released by the hypothalamus that stimulates the pituitary gland to secrete thyroid-stimulating hormone (TSH).

Thyroxine—the primary hormone produced by the thyroid gland. Naturally formed from iodine atoms, this hormone circulates through the body primarily bound to carrier proteins. It functions to regulate metabolism. It is available in animal and synthetic forms as replacement when the thyroid produces little or no thyroxine itself.

Thyroxine binding globulin (TBG)—the major thyroid hormone transport protein in human serum.

Thyroxine binding proteins (TBP)—three serum proteins with binding affinities for T4 and T3: thyroxine binding globulin (TBG), prealbumin, and albumin.

Tissue—a group of cells organized to perform a specialized function.

TSH (thyroid stimulating hormone)—a pituitary hormone (thyrotropin) that promotes growth of the thyroid gland and stimulates the thyroid gland to secret hormones.

TSH test—a test to measure the amount of thyroid-stimulating hormone (TSH) in the bloodstream.

Trachea—the windpipe.

Triiodothyronine (T3)—a hormone produced by the thyroid gland, as well as by the breakdown of thyroxine (T4). Sometimes a person cannot do this adequately and must take a synthetic form of T3.

Tumor—an uncontrolled progressive growth of cells resulting from excessive cell division. Also called neoplasm.

T-uptake—a measurement of the total binding capacity of the thyroxine binding proteins for thyroid hormones.

Turner's Syndrome—a rare genetic disorder resulting in a complete or partial absence of one of the two X chromosomes in the female, inhibiting normal sexual development and causing sterility.

Ultrasound—an imaging technique used to obtain pictures by bouncing sound waves off an object.

Vitiligo—a skin condition characterized by white patches of skin resulting from loss of pigment. Melanin, the pigment that determines skin color, is produced in cells called melanocytes. Vitiligo occurs when melanocytes die or are unable to produce melanin.

Index

adrenal glands, 47, 78–80, 95

alternative therapies, alternative therapists, 182–83, 219–20, 226

antidepressants, xiv, 12, 15, 70, 151, 157, 160
  diagnosing hypothyroidism and, 25–26, 30, 32
  tricyclic, 55, 67, 78, 112

atrophic thyroiditis, 87, 95

autoimmune hypothyroidism, 112, 120, 122–23, 131

autoimmune thyroiditis, 87, 89, 91–96, 99–100, 115, 156

autoimmunity, autoimmune problems, 83, 89–96, 99–101, 158, 190
  adolescence and, 148–49, 151
  chart on, 100–101
  childhood hypothyroidism and, 140–41
  genetics in, 91–92, 99
  hypothyroid work sheet and, 106–7
  mini-lesson on, 89–91
  pregnancy and, 122–23

  see also Hashimoto's autoimmune thyroiditis

beans, 201–4, 208–9

beef, 187, 201, 204

behavior and learning problems, 53, 114–15, 133, 150
  and childhood hypothyroidism, 139, 141, 144–45
  and environmental toxins, 186–88, 192
  and hypothyroidism in infants, 129–30

bones, 56, 137, 189
  menopause and, 164, 168–70, 172

breakfasts, 200, 203–6

breast-feeding concerns, 132

calcium supplements, 56, 170–71, 215

cardiac problems, 8, 33, 55, 105, 113, 120, 130, 135, 159, 189
  elderly and, 173–77
  explanations for, 74–75
  fats and, 71–72

cardiac problems (*cont.*)
  menopause and, 164, 167–70, 172
  treating hypothyroidism and, 53–54
chicken, 187, 200–201, 203–4, 210, 219
children:
  environmental toxins and, 186–87,
    191–92
  hypothyroidism in, 19, 117–18, 139–46
chronic fatigue syndrome (CFS), 65–66, 80
congenital hypothyroidism, 78, 88, 134–39,
    144

dairy products, 187, 201, 203–4, 210, 218
DDT, 186, 214
depression, 67–70, 82, 85, 88, 105, 131,
    148–49, 188, 219, 222
  adolescence and, 149, 151
  bibliographic extracts on, 112–15
  men and, 157, 160
  menopause and, 164, 170, 172
  in SAD, 67–69
de Quervain's thyroiditis, 95–96
diabetes, 65, 71–72, 85, 93, 95, 99–100,
    107, 131, 158, 160, 196
dinners, 200, 203–4, 208–10
doctors, finding, 223–26

eggs, 201, 203–6
elderly, 33, 88, 111, 173–79, 186
  hypothyroidism in, 20–21, 97, 118,
    175–79
environmental toxins, 89, 92, 99, 103,
    185–92
estrogen, estrogens, 20, 29, 55, 63, 80, 82,
    86, 121, 212–13
  adolescence and, 148–49
  autoimmune problems and, 92–94
  environmental toxins and, 186, 188–90
  menopause and, 161–70
exercise, 23, 29, 57, 64–66, 69, 75, 159,
    174, 182
  fats and, 71–72
  menopause and, 162, 164, 170–71
  tips from Dr. Blanchard's patients on,
    216–19
  weight gain and, 194–96

family histories, xv–xvi, 12, 19–20, 133,
    136, 158
  adolescence and, 148, 150–51
  autoimmune problems and, 92, 99

childhood hypothyroidism and, 140–41
diagnosing hypothyroidism and, 30, 103,
    108–9
fat, fats, 71–75, 106, 111, 169, 187,
    195–96, 200, 202, 221–22
fatigue, xiv–xvi, 4, 8–9, 14, 18, 25, 37–38,
    70, 77, 88, 95, 98, 115, 121, 131,
    138, 154, 157, 188, 193, 195, 199
  adolescence and, 147–50
  CFS and, 65–66, 80
  childhood hypothyroidism and, 139, 143
  elderly and, 173, 175
  in fibromyalgia, 62–63, 65
  menopause and, 161, 163, 170, 172
  pregnancy and, 127, 129–30
  treating hypothyroidism and, 58, 72–73
fertility, 3, 20, 35, 80, 86, 97, 105, 119–20,
    122–23, 148, 152, 190, 193
fibromyalgia, 62–67, 85, 89, 99, 219
fish, 187–88, 201, 203–4, 207, 209–10,
    214–15, 219
fluoride, 186, 191–92
fruits and vegetables, 187, 201–5, 207, 211,
    213, 219

gastrointestinal problems, 4, 10, 14, 19,
    105, 125, 138
  hypothyroid mechanism of, 83–84, 86
  menopause and, 170, 172
genetics, 88–89, 91–92, 99, 133, 136
goiters, 27, 36, 94–95, 101–2, 112, 139,
    156, 213
  adolescence and, 149, 151–52
  environmental toxins and, 191–92
Graves' disease, xvi, 28, 80, 94, 96, 98, 112,
    131, 165, 191
growth rates, 140–41, 149–50

hair loss, xv–xvi, 4, 119, 159, 188, 193,
    195
  diagnosing hypothyroidism and, 29–30,
    104
  hypothyroid mechanism of, 81–82, 85
  menopause and, 161–62, 172
Hashimoto's autoimmune thyroiditis, 9–10,
    28, 48, 59, 80, 82–83, 86–87, 89,
    91–96, 120, 122–23, 141, 175, 191
headaches, 4, 9, 14, 18–19, 88, 104, 147,
    149, 188, 193
  menopause and, 165–66, 170, 172

high blood pressure, 74–75, 105, 127–28, 176
holistic habits, 212–15
homeopathy, 24, 182, 220
hydrotherapy, 220
hyperthyroidism, 12, 47, 49, 57, 87, 94–95, 113, 131, 192, 195, 197
hypothyroidism:
  causes of, 9, 37, 47, 60, 79, 87–89, 91–99, 102, 111–12, 135–36, 143, 174, 185, 190–91, 213
  diagnosis of, xi, xiii–xvi, xviii, 5–6, 8–9, 11–16, 19–20, 22–33, 50–51, 53–54, 57, 87, 103–9, 117–19, 124, 131, 137, 140, 143–44, 149–52, 158–59, 165, 171, 174–75, 178–79, 181, 193, 223–24
  early stages of, 45–46
  myths about, xi, xvi
  symptoms of, xiii–xvi, 3–10, 12, 14–16, 18–27, 29–30, 32–33, 35, 37–38, 43, 48, 50, 52–54, 57–58, 60–67, 69, 72, 75–78, 80–86, 88, 92, 94–96, 98, 103–6, 111, 113–15, 117, 119–20, 122, 125, 128–33, 136–39, 141–45, 147–52, 154, 156–59, 164–65, 170–72, 175–76, 178–79, 182, 188, 224–25
  treatment of, xi, xiii–xviii, 5–13, 15–24, 26, 29–30, 32–35, 38–45, 48–61, 63–64, 67–69, 72–73, 77–78, 80, 84, 88, 94–95, 98, 111, 117–20, 123–30, 132, 134–36, 138–45, 147–48, 152, 154, 158–60, 165, 169, 171, 174–75, 181–82, 223–24, 226
  work sheet on, 103–9

infants, 88, 129–30, 134–39, 186, 189
infection, infections, 66, 80, 86, 92, 158, 164, 175, 177
insulin, 54, 65, 72–73, 216
insulin resistance, 159, 196
iodine, 35–36, 189, 213
  deficiency of, 101–2, 129
  radioactive, 88, 95–96, 98, 165
iron supplements, 55–56, 124
irritable bowel syndrome (IBS), 66, 83–84, 86, 89, 99–100, 105

levothyroxine, 9–10, 39–40, 43
libido, xv, 54, 105, 148, 190

hypothyroid mechanism of, 82, 86
men and, 157–60
menopause and, 161–62, 172
lunches, 200, 203–4, 206–7

massage, 221
medications, xiii–xvii, 6–13, 15–20, 22–23, 39–43, 66–70, 80, 88–89, 117–21, 123–30
  adolescence and, 151–52
  for autoimmune problems, 100–101
  childhood hypothyroidism and, 141–45
  compounding of, 40–42, 52, 59
  congenital hypothyroidism and, 136, 138–39
  for depression/SAD, 67–69
  diagnosing hypothyroidism and, 12–13, 15, 25–26, 30, 32–33, 103, 107
  dosages of, 7, 10, 17–18, 22, 30, 34, 39–40, 43, 49–54, 56–60, 67–69, 77, 95, 99, 117, 120–21, 124–29, 132, 138–39, 143–45, 153–55, 157, 162, 166, 170, 173–75, 178–79, 181, 193–99, 215, 224–25
  elderly and, 173–79
  for fibromyalgia, 66–67
  finding doctors and, 223–25
  holistic habits and, 213, 215
  interactions of, 54–55, 124–25, 215
  men and, 157–58, 160
  menopause and, 162, 165–71
  mental fogginess and, 77–78
  nutrition and, 199, 201
  PMS and, 153–54
  side effects of, 10, 17, 49, 54–55, 57, 59, 70, 101, 153
  weight gain and, 193–98
  see also antidepressants
men, 54, 156–60, 175
menopause, 3, 20, 23, 54, 63, 80, 105, 118, 161–72, 189
menstruation, 3–4, 120–22, 218, 220
  adolescence and, 147–50, 152
  gastrointestinal problems and, 84
  menopause and, 163, 165, 169
mental fogginess, 5, 9–10, 18, 29, 66, 69–71, 75–78, 85, 98, 105, 130, 139, 150, 172–73, 175, 195
mercury contamination, 188, 214–15
mild (subclinical) hypothyroidism, 87, 96–97, 111, 119–21, 123

mild hypothyroidism (*cont.*)
  in elderly, 175–76, 178
moisturizers, 215
mood swings, 115, 139, 151, 163, 172
multiple sclerosis (MS), 100, 107, 156–57
muscles and joints, 4, 69, 79, 95, 131, 138,
    149, 195–96, 218
  and elderly, 173, 175
  in fibromyalgia, 62–63, 66–67
  and hypothyroid mechanisms, 84–85
  and hypothyroid work sheet, 104–5
  and menopause, 164, 170, 172
  and nutrition, 199–200
  and symptoms of hypothyroidism, 62–67
myasthenia gravis, 100, 107
myxedema coma, 177

nail brittleness, 81, 85, 104
natural thyroid extract (Armour), 9–10,
    17–18, 64, 224
  answers to questions about, 59–60
  elderly and, 173–74
  pregnancy and, 120, 128
  treating hypothyroidism and, 42–43, 48,
    52–54, 59–60, 120, 128
nutrition, 21, 23, 48, 89, 102, 107, 159,
    169–70, 178, 198–214
  environmental toxins and, 187–90
  holistic habits and, 212–14
  metabolism and, 199–203
  Thyroid Wellness Diet and, 182, 203–11
  tips from Dr. Blanchard's patients on,
    216, 218–19
  and variety of foods, 202–3
  weight gain and, 194, 196, 198
nutritional supplements, 182, 221–22
nuts, 202–3, 209–10

phytoestrogens, 188–90, 212–14
  menopause and, 169–70
postpartum thyroiditis, 53, 130–32
pregnancy, 20, 23, 33, 78, 88–89, 112–13,
    117, 119–31, 136
  autoimmune problems and, 122–23
  dosing guidelines during, 128–29
  seasonal issues and, 125–29
  thyroid hormones and, 120, 124–25,
    127–29
  treating hypothyroidism and, 53, 127–29
  TSH tests and, 120–21, 123, 125
pregnancy-induced thyroiditis, 97

premenstrual syndrome (PMS), xiv–xv, 4,
    19, 21, 38, 45, 53, 80, 84, 86, 88,
    105, 120–21, 133, 139, 147, 152–55
puberty, 3, 23, 88, 130
  hypothyroidism in, 19–20, 118, 147–52

recipes, 205–11
rheumatoid arthritis, 99–100, 107, 158
Riedel's thyroiditis, 87, 95

S-adenosylmethionine (SAMe), 219
safer sex, 214
salt, 213
scleroderma, 101
seasonal affective disorder (SAD), 67–69,
    105
seasonal conditions, 21, 23, 53, 57–58, 85,
    97, 177
  pregnancy and, 125–29
selenium, 47–48, 182, 222
silent thyroiditis, 96
Sjögren's syndrome, 82, 101, 107
skin problems, 4, 9–10, 18, 29, 38, 67,
    81–82, 84–85, 104, 139, 143, 164,
    172, 175
sleep problems, 4, 9–10, 62–67, 79, 104,
    149, 194–96
  menopause and, 161, 163, 172
smoking, 108, 112–13, 190–91
snacks, 204, 211, 218–19
soy foods, 169, 189–90, 201, 212–13, 219
stress, 24, 78–80, 106, 177, 220
  autoimmune problems and, 92
  men and, 158–59
surgically induced hypothyroidism, 88, 98
systemic lupus erythematosus, 99, 101,
    106–7, 156, 158

thyroid:
  functions of, 19, 35–37, 45
  size and shape of, 35
thyroid cancer, 98–99, 115, 158
thyroid-friendly foods, 200–202
thyroid hormones, 4–5, 8, 10, 20–21,
    35–48, 62, 69, 99, 101, 120–21, 132
  adolescence and, 148, 151
  answers to questions about treatment
    with, 55–60
  childhood hypothyroidism and, 143–44
  fats and, 71–72
  infancy and, 134–39

medication interactions with, 54–55
men and, 156–57
menopause and, 164–66, 169
mental fogginess and, 75–76, 85
PMS and, 153–55
pregnancy and, 120, 124–25, 127–29
thyroid nodules, 98–99, 158
thyroid stimulating hormone (TSH), 9, 32,
    63, 68, 71, 84, 88, 96–97, 99, 132
    in autoimmune problems, 91, 93
    bibliographic extracts on, 110–11, 115
    elderly and, 175, 177–79
    infancy and, 134, 137
    menopause and, 162, 165
    and problems converting T4 to T3,
        46–47
    supply and demand for, 37–38
    treating hypothyroidism and, 51, 57–58,
        72
    weight gain and, 195, 197–98
Thyroid Wellness Diet, 182, 203–11
thyroxine (T4), xiii–xiv, xvii, 5–7, 9–11,
    15–18, 22–23, 32–36, 51–60, 71–72,
    74, 79, 84–85, 88–89, 95–96, 102,
    187, 213, 223
    answers to questions about, 56–60
    in autoimmune problems, 89, 91–92,
        94
    bibliographic extracts on, 110–11, 115
    childhood hypothyroidism, 143–45
    for depression/SAD, 67–68
    diagnosing hypothyroidism and, 28–29,
        32–33
    in early stages of hypothyroidism, 45–46
    elderly and, 173–74, 177–79
    fibromyalgia and, 63–65
    and hypothyroidism in infants, 129,
        136–38
    men and, 157–58
    menopause and, 162, 165–66, 170–71
    mental fogginess and, 77–78, 85
    phytoestrogens and, 189–90
    PMS and, 153–55
    pregnancy and, 120, 124, 128–29
    problems with convert it to T3, 45–48,
        65, 85, 89
    supply and demand for, 38–39
    treating hypothyroidism and, 34–35,
        39–40, 43–45, 51–54, 56–60, 84, 95,
        111, 117–20, 124, 128–29, 165, 181
    weight gain and, 193–95, 197

traditional Chinese medicine, 221
treatment-induced hypothyroidism, 88, 98
triiodothyronine (T3), xvii, 5, 7–8, 16–18,
    22–23, 34–54, 63–69, 71–72, 74,
    77–79, 84–85, 102, 144, 187, 213,
    222, 224
    answers to questions about, 56–60
    in autoimmune problems, 89, 91–92, 94
    bibliographic extracts on, 111–12,
        114–15
    depression and, 68–69
    diagnosing hypothyroidism and, 28–29,
        32
    in early stages of hypothyroidism, 45–46
    elderly and, 173–75, 177–78
    fibromyalgia and, 63–67
    men and, 157–58
    menopause and, 162, 165–66, 170–71
    mental fogginess and, 77–78, 85
    phytoestrogens and, 189–90
    PMS and, 154–55
    pregnancy and, 120, 124, 127–29
    problems converting T4 to, 45–48, 65,
        85, 89
    reverse, 36, 43
    supply and demand for, 37–39
    treating hypothyroidism and, 34–35,
        39–45, 48–54, 56–60, 72, 84, 95,
        117–18, 120, 124, 127–29, 165, 181
    weight gain and, 193–95, 198
TSH tests, xi, xiv–xvi, 7, 11–15, 20–22, 98,
    147–48
    answers to questions about, 57–58
    childhood hypothyroidism and, 139–40,
        145
    congenital hypothyroidism and, 136–37
    diagnosing hypothyroidism and, 25–26,
        28–33
    finding doctors and, 223–25
    men and, 157–58
    normal range for, 12, 14, 26, 28–32,
        46–48, 51, 54, 57, 125–26, 148,
        157–58, 165, 170, 224
    PMS and, 154–55
    pregnancy and, 120–21, 123, 125
    treating hypothyroidism and, 34, 38, 119
turkey, 201, 203–4, 218–19
Two-Week Diagnostic Trial, 50–51,
    117–18, 143–44, 151, 178–79

vitamins, 56, 124, 182, 215, 221

water, 202, 213, 215
weight gain, xiv, xvi, 4, 8–9, 21, 70–73, 75,
　　84, 95, 98, 128, 138–39, 154, 193–98
　causes of, 64–65, 85
　childhood hypothyroidism and, 139, 143
　control of, 23, 64
　diagnosing hypothyroidism and, 29–30
　elderly and, 173–74
　men and, 157, 159

menopause and, 164, 172
rebound effect and, 197–98
T4 and, 193–95, 197
treating hypothyroidism and, 58, 72
weight loss, 199–200, 216–18

xenoestrogens, 186–87, 214–15

yoga, 9–10, 24, 170, 196, 217–18

About the Authors

KENNETH R. BLANCHARD M.D., Ph.D., is an endocrinologist certified by the American Board of Internal Medicine and the American Board of Endocrinology and Metabolism. He studied as an undergraduate at MIT, received a Ph.D. in chemistry from Princeton University, and completed his medical studies at Cornell University Medical College. Dr. Blanchard completed his residency at New York–Memorial Hospital in New York City and his Fellowship in Endocrinology at Boston VA Hospital. His private practice in Newton-Wellesley, Massachusetts, consumes most of his time, although he addresses many types of groups on the topic of hypothyroidism and is considered an authority on the subject. His reputation for successful treatment of hypothyroidism draws an international patient base. He participates in health symposiums for lay audiences and for professionals and has appeared on local television health programs. He developed his unique, successful approach to hypothyroidism based on twenty-five years of observations, cautious empirical treatment, and mounting clinical evidence. Dr. Blanchard is the father of two children and lives in Waban, Massachusetts, with his wife, Rita.

MARIETTA ABRAMS BRILL is a freelance writer with three health books to her credit: *Living with Lupus* (Putnam, 1994), *The Headache Alternative* (Dell, 1996), and *The Harvard Medical School Family Health Guide* (primary writer; Simon & Schuster, 1999). She and her family split their time between New York City and Woodstock, New York.